Fitness After Forty

Fitness After Forty

Hal Higdon

Published by
World Publications

Recommended Reading:
Runner's World Magazine, $9.50/year
Write for a free catalog of publications
and supplies for runners and other athletes.

© 1977 by
World Publications
P.O. Box 366, Mountain View, CA 94042

No information in this book may be reprinted in any
form without permission from the publisher.

Library of Congress 77-783-34
ISBN 0-89037-076 (Hb) -077-X (Ppb)

OTHER BOOKS BY HAL HIGDON

The Union vs. Dr. Mudd
Pro Football USA
The Business Healers
Finding the Groove
Find the Key Man
On the Run from Dogs and People
The Crime of the Century
Summer of Triumph

FOR CHILDREN

Heroes of the Olympics
The Horse that Played Center Field
Thirty Days in May
Champions of the Tennis Courts
The Electronic Olympics
Six Seconds to Glory
The Last Series
Showdown at Daytona

Contents

Introduction 2

PART ONE: IN SEARCH OF LIFE 7
  1. The Rise and Fall of the Human Empire 8
  2. A Disneyland for Joggers 23
  3. The Quest for a Coronary-Prone Characteristic 42
  4. On the Edge of His Chair 58
  5. Targets 68

PART TWO: ATHLETICS FOR OLDSTERS 85
  6. "They're Not Runners; They're Too Old" 86
  7. Death of a Distance Runner 102
  8. What Is Your True Athletic Potential? 122

PART THREE: FOOD AND FITNESS 131
  9. The Battle of the Bulge 132
 10. The Miracle Diet Doctor of the Mountains 142
 11. Food for Athletes 157

PART FOUR: TRAINING FOR A LIFETIME 175
 12. Renaissance Sportsman 176
 13. The Pain of P.E. 190
 14. What Sports Are Best for Fitness? 196
 15. The Semi-Obligatory Physical Examination Disclaimer . 224
 16. Keeping It Up 237

Epilogue: How to Live to Be 99 247

Introduction

Perhaps at no other time in history has the need for exercise been so great. Man once stayed fit through hard work. But by the 20th century, automation and other technological advances had converted him into a sedentary being. Traveling by automobile became a way of life. Television locked him into his living room. Suburbs no longer were built with sidewalks, under the assumption that nobody walks any more.

"Inactivity," Theodore L. Klumpp, M.D., once claimed, "is one of the chief saboteurs of health. We don't wear out; we rust out."

In the United States, more than one million people die of cardiovascular diseases each year. According to the American Heart Association, 54% of the deaths occurring in the United States during 1974 were due to this cause.

Dr. Paul Dudley White, President Eisenhower's physician, once stated, "The greatest challenge of public and private health today, and the most neglected, is that of physical fitness in middle age. It transcends, I believe, the problems of health of both youth and senility. The laudable goal of improving the physical (and mental) health of our youth should have no age limit at any decade, but it ought to continue on where it is needed most all through life."

In recent years, many government officials and health authorities have stressed the need for physical fitness. And fitness is particularly needed by people near the age of 40, who suddenly become aware of their own mortality. But what exactly is "fitness"?

To many people, fitness merely means strength. Many of the best-selling exercise books in the 1960s, after President Kennedy made fitness seem respectable, revolved around calisthenic programs. Actually, physical fitness consists of more than strength. It includes endurance. In fact, endurance is especially important.

Physical fitness allows you (your abilities) to work without undue fatigue, to retain enough energy to enjoy hobbies and recreational activities, and to make optimal use of your body. Fitness means being capable of meeting unexpected emergencies. Fitness not only applies to the muscular athlete; it includes the handicapped person who uses his body fully. It not only applies to youthful Olympians, but also to men and women past retirement age who still can keep active. Fitness also includes your health, your ability to fight infection and your freedom from disease.

You might compare a physically fit person to a well-tuned automotive engine. The engine may run quietly while it is idling, yet be ready to deliver a burst of power once the driver steps on the gas.

"Muscles are the motors of the human body," Dr. Klumpp has said. "Their efficiency and the ease and grace with which they perform depend on their tone."

What are some of the benefits of fitness?

First, the body contains more than 600 muscles which make possible every movement. These muscles perform many activities. They pass food along the digestive tract, maintain posture, suck air into the lungs and tighten blood vessels to elevate the blood pressure when more pressure is needed in an emergency. The heart itself is a muscular pump which can only operate efficiently if it is exercised regularly.

Exercise does many things:

1. *Exercise stimulates circulation.* When you exercise your

muscles, your circulation increases. Your heart beats stronger to furnish more oxygen to the muscles and remove waste material. As your cells receive oxygen faster, you begin to feel better. Also, the more often your heart and circulatory system move blood to active regions of the body, the more efficient they become.

2. Exercise builds endurance. A fit person can perform the same movements as a flabby or a weak one—with less effort and over a longer period of time. The old axiom says, "Practice makes perfect." This is true in fitness, too.

3. Exercise helps you relax. It provides a good antidote for nervous tension. Exercise is one of the best means for relaxation since general muscular fatigue is conducive to physical and mental rest, and sleep.

Dr. White claimed, "You will not need tranquilizers or hypnotics if you take a long walk in the evening, or run a mile or two if you are young enough. You will not need sedatives. Nature will supply you with pleasant sleeping."

I have only one quarrel with this statement by Dr. White, made nearly two decades ago. It is his reference to running a mile, only "if you are young enough." What is young enough? Being young and capable of running a mile once meant only individuals in their teens and 20s, maybe 30s. Until recently, very few people continued running past the age of 40. Very few people attempted to compete in any sport.

But during the summer of 1975 at the First World Masters Track and Field Championships in Toronto, Canada (a series of athletic competitions limited to men and women age 40 and up), I witnessed an exhibition race at 200 meters among three sprinters aged 81, 88 and 90. Youth prevailed as the youngest, Fritz Schreiber of Sweden, beat Duncan MacLean of Scotland and Charles Speechley of England. It was the most exciting race of the week-long meeting.

The time of the fastest of the trio was nearly twice what might be expected from teenage sprinters in the Olympic Games. But most people would consider being able to move at that age, much less run, an accomplishment. The oldest of the trio seemed to be the sprightliest: MacLean, who at one time in his long life served as understudy for Scottish performer Harry Loder.

"I've been running all my life," MacLean claimed. "I've had a wonderful life, but I'm not finished yet. You have to keep moving about. Otherwise, when you're as old as I am, you relax too much."

Not everyone can expect to match Duncan MacLean's accomplishments at age 90. Insurance company actuarial tables indicate that only a few of us even will reach that age. But there has been a recent upsurge of athletics for oldsters. Much of it has come in age-group competition in which athletes are matched against others their age. However, a few senior citizen sportsmen still compete successfully against younger persons.

Jack Foster of New Zealand competed in the 1976 Olympics in Montreal at age 44 and ran near the front of the marathon for much of the race, eventually finishing 17th out of 67 of the most select competitors in that event in the world.

In other sports, Hoyt Wilhelm pitched successfully in the major leagues until age 49. George Blanda was into his 50s before finally retiring from professional football as a quarterback and placekicker. Pancho Gonzales in tennis and Arnold Palmer in golf continue to achieve success in their sports into their 40s. Bobby Riggs waited until age 55 to achieve fame and fortune in tennis.

But for every Foster or Blanda or Riggs in the limelight of the public arena, thousands of other men and women over 40 are awakening to the fact that their bodies need not deteriorate with age—or, if they inevitably must deteriorate, it need not happen as rapidly as we have been led to assume by well-meaning physicians who caution us to take it easy in middle age and beyond.

Many people today are interested in fitness after 40. These are individuals who have become concerned about their diets, who have shifted to a more moderate life style, who have decided that sports are not just something you watch on television Sunday afternoons. On Sundays, they are the ones out jogging in the woods, cycling down the roads, swimming at the local pool, or playing racquetball or tennis on a nearby court. To them, the future Duncan MacLeans of the world, this book is dedicated.

Hal Higdon
Michigan City, Ind.
March, 1977

Part One:
IN SEARCH OF LIFE

1
The Rise and Fall Of the Human Empire

Plato wrote about human development four centuries before Christ: "Though indeed we may pretend that a person lives and is the same from birth until death, in actual fact he never is exactly in the same condition with the same properties, since everything in him is in a constant state of decay and renewal—his hair, his flesh, his warmth, his blood and, in short, his whole body; and not only his body, but his soul, his habits, manners and customs, his opinions, wants and desires... all are in a constant state of flux, waxing and waning all the time."

The way in which the human body develops is a complex process. Man begins life in his mother's womb: an ovum (egg) fertilized by a single sperm cell from the father. The ovum begins to grow in the first few weeks. Before much differentiation begins, there are only germ layers: the mesoderm, from which comes the muscles and connective tissues; the ectoderm, from which comes the skin and nervous system; the endoderm, from which will be formed the gastrointestinal tract.

Eighteen days after fertilization, the ectoderm thickens to become the neural plate. The limbs begin, looking like small buds on the surface of the embryo. In the fourth week comes the beginnings of the eyes, ears and nose. By the end of that week, the head appears with forebrain, midbrain and hindbrain differentiated. The main organ systems have become established. Through the sixth week, the human embryo differs little from that of other mammals. By eight weeks, however, the head enlarges as the brain develops, and the embryo starts to look human. External genitals appear.

The heart, so central to human life, starts beating regularly by four weeks, takes shape by six and becomes four-chambered by 14. Blood formation in the marrow will have begun at 12 weeks. The lungs also take shape at 12 weeks, with elastic fibers appearing in them in 16. At about this time, ossification begins as bones, previously like cartilage, obtain calcium and phosphorous. Fingers and toes now have nails. The external genitals exhibit definite signs of sex.

The skin is wrinkled but becomes less transparent. It becomes covered with down. Hair grows on the head. Between 20 and 24 weeks of development, fat starts to become deposited beneath the skin, and some of the wrinkles start smoothing out. By 28 weeks, the retinal layers are complete, and the eyes can perceive light. A child born at this stage of development can move his limbs energetically and cry in a weak voice.

The body continues to grow in the next half-dozen weeks, and by about 40 weeks—or the ninth month of pregnancy—the miracle of birth occurs. The child is thrust from the womb—sometimes is pulled or torn from the womb—into a cold, hostile and cruel environment which will test his ability to survive.

But the newborn child has not yet finished growing, although after the first year growth will slow from its previous fetal rate. If a child continued growing at that rate, he would stand 20 feet tall by age 10.

The brain develops fastest. Weighing 0.8 pound at birth, it will reach 2.2 pounds by one year. By puberty, the brain, at its maximum growth, will be only 0.7 pound heavier (or 2.9 pounds). The skull bones remain relatively soft at birth, often molded somewhat by their passage through the birth channel. By one year, the skull becomes symmetrical. An increase of fat for insulation occurs during this first year then gradually disappears as the child continues to grow.

The nervous system is nearly complete at birth. A baby is born with perhaps 10 billion neurons, from which the nervous system is made, and will add no more after the first three months. As the child develops, these neurons grow, add new glial cells and develop myelination (fatty insulating sheaths on the neuron fibers — in other words, new connections).

Of all the organs of the body, the heart, in its growth rate, most closely parallels the growth of the entire body (with the liver a close second). Although the cardiovascular system is fully developed at birth, it must accommodate itself to circulation demands different from those in the uterus.

Baby teeth show development beginning in the womb. Primary teeth begin to develop six months after birth. At age six, the baby teeth start to drop out, being replaced by the permanent teeth, all of which are in place by 12 years. Puberty, the final sexual development, usually begins with girls after age 10 and with boys after age 12. There is one last growth spurt before a hormone from the pituitary gland causes the bones the fuse, usually around 16 in females and 18 in males. The body will grow no taller. The age at which eyes achieve their maturity also differs: around 20 for women, 26 for men. Most men achieve their physiological maturity by age 26. Women achieve theirs somewhat earlier. The bone and muscle structure reach the point of maximum efficiency.

Age 26 is the point — theoretical at least — when the human body has reached its prime, the time at which athletes reach their peak. This point starts the decline, a steady deterioration of the body systems which eventually results in so-called "old age" and death. The slope of the decline is difficult to recognize at first, but it soon turns more steeply downward. It takes a quarter-century for the body to develop to its fullest potential, and it takes approximately two more quarter-centuries (according to current actuarial tables) for that body to deteriorate to the point where it no longer functions.

Of course, not all systems of the body reach maturity at the same time and not all decay at the same rate. For some systems, decay may begin even before maturity. A smoking mother poisons her unborn child with nicotine even before his first breath. Children of drug-addict mothers are born with signs of addiction. Decay in the teeth may begin almost as soon as those teeth appear, depending on the care given them. Obese children, who overeat even before becoming teenagers, may never reach their potential peak of physical health.

Autopsies of young American soldiers killed during the Korean War showed many with atherosclerotic deposits already beginning to clog their arteries, the result of poor diet and inadequate exercise. Fatty deposits were present in the arterial walls of 77% of these men averaging age 22. Ten per cent of those autopsied had occlusions of more than 70% in one or more of their arteries! Their bodies were deteriorating while still developing.

Yet others, who have reached their theoretical peak as physical beings, may not necessarily decline immediately. Patterns differ between individuals and within individuals.

"The body continues to develop throughout life," suggests Jay Berkelhamer, M.D., a pediatrician with the University of Chicago Hospitals. "Although you reach some point in time when all systems start to degenerate, it is arbitrary when that occurs. It probably occurs between 25 and 30 years of life, but there also must be a period when you can maintain your physical capabilities, and that could extend for a long time."

Some hint as to when that time occurs can be gleaned by examining the records of athletes, the point at which peak performances occur in different sports. Swimmers mature very early, reaching top levels in their early teens. Yet few of them continue to improve beyond their late teens. Sprinters in track achieve peak performances at age 22; milers at age 25; middle-distance runners at age 27, and long-distance runners at age 29. Only rare athletes succeed in Olympic competition into their 30s.

The peak year for most baseball players seems to be age 28 or 29. In addition to raw physical ability, experience or maturity often is a factor and one difficult to measure. In many team sports, the position a person plays may affect his longevity. In professional basketball, forwards, who must jump as well as shoot, fade quicker than guards who rely more on intelligent playmaking. However, a center, whose main attribute is height and weight, may outlast everybody.

In football, the longevity of running backs (which is influenced by the pounding they take from tacklers) parallels that of sprinters in track. Linemen last longer since strength and size, plus experience, may be as important as mobility for some of them. Defensive linemen, who hit more often than get hit, last longer than offensive linemen, just as defensive backs outlast receivers. The oldest football players, however, frequently are quarterbacks for whom intelligence and experience may be even more important ingredients in their success than strong throwing arms. For this same reason, relief pitchers outlast starting pitchers, or others on their baseball club.

By age 30, boxers have begun to lose the hand-eye coordination that contributed to their success. The same is true with tennis players. Jockeys find they have difficulty maintaining their weight level near the 100 pounds necessary to obtain good rides. But at this age, Indianapolis race drivers have just begun to develop the experience necessary to drive skillfully as well as fast and, most important, the contacts with sponsors and owners to give them the best equipment. Ultra-marathon runners (those racing in events such as 50 miles) have just begun to accumulate a sufficient background of training miles that will permit them to go far as well as fast.

For athletes in contact sports, their longevity may depend in part upon the amount of battering their body receives. According to Jack Bell of the American Medical Association's Committee on the Medical Aspects of Sports, "An older player gets burned out partly because he is less agile, but previous injuries may contribute to his lack of agility."

When Johnny Unitas retired as quarterback after a professional career that spanned two decades, he commented, "They tell you that things change at 40, but they don't tell you how much."

For many athletes, particularly in non-contact sports, the slide downward may be as much psychological as physiological. A teenage swimmer abandons the water not from a decline in abilities but from a decline in interest. It no longer seems important to train two-hour sessions, twice a day, to satisfy an urge for medals, trophies and victories. Track athletes discover they must compete with increasing waves of younger, bigger, better fed, better trained runners, who continue to push records ever downward beyond their elders' capabilities. Athletes in football, basketball and baseball graduate from high school or college and, unless gifted enough to earn a professional contract, find a lack of organized teams for which they can play. There is no Little League, or its equivalent, for people in their 20s.

Female athletes become interested in males, get married and become pregnant (not necessarily in that order). Male athletes (and increasing numbers of females) find that career advancement conflicts with athletic goals. Many athletes—in fact, *most* athletes—retire before even nearing their physical prime. Others retire despite the fact they could have maintained their prime much longer than they desired.

"Our concepts of aging and athletics are going to change," says Thomas Bassler, M.D., a Los Angeles-area physician and president of the American Medical Joggers Association. "We may find out that the peak in performance may be around 29, but the slope afterwards is not as steep as we think it may be."

Some understanding of the effect of aging on the performances of athletes, *if* they continued to condition themselves beyond the theoretical point of peak performance, can be learned by examining the development of singers.

According to Wilma Osheim, a Chicago-area voice teacher, "In adolescence, when voices mature, boys and girls have trouble singing because their vocal cords have thickened and they have not yet learned to support the new voice. Their strength seems to go into maturing the rest of the body, and the result is a breathy tone, especially for girls."

Osheim says several things are needed for good singing: abdominal strength, maturity of vocal cords in the larynx, and mental and emotional maturity. A coloratura, the highest voice range for women, matures between the ages of 21 and 25. The lower the voice, the longer before it reaches maturity. For a mezzo or contralto, maturity comes between 30 and 35. But unlike the apparent pattern in sports, reaching a peak in singing does not necessarily mean that decline will begin. A good singer often has 20 or 30 "peak" years.

"If the voice is used properly," Osheim insists, "a person can sing in top form until the late 60s or even early 70s." The decline finally comes when muscles lose elasticity and general body strength declines. Coordination of muscles is as important in singing as in athletics, despite lessened intensity.

Other parallels exist between singing and athletics. Patrice Munsel, the famous coloratura, sang at the Metropolitan Opera between ages 18 and 20, a very rare occurrence. She burned out early because she taxed her voice too much, too soon. Another famous opera singer once said, when asked the secret of his success, that he only sang what he could do well, and nothing else. A young person who forces himself to sing music too difficult can ruin his voice due to muscle strain. Rock singers sometimes destroy their voices within a few years because, being untrained, they fail to support their voices with proper breathing. Nodes can develop on vocal cords from continued abuse. The problems faced by singers seemingly resemble those faced by fastball pitchers, who develop sore arms, or tennis players with dreaded "tennis elbow."

The ability of a coloratura to maintain her singing ability is not easily measured statistically, nor can her performance at one age be accurately compared with that at another age. Even the won-lost records of baseball pitchers and tennis players are affected by the skills of their opponents. Only in a few sports, where stopwatches accurately measure performance, can reasonably precise determinations be made on the effort aging has on a person's ability to compete.

One such sport is swimming, where Ransom J. Arthur, M.D., a professor at UCLA's Neuro-Psychiatric Institute and Richard H. Rahe of the Naval Health Research Center in San Diego determined the relative effects of aging. Dr. Arthur, age 52, competes in Masters swim competitions (for athletes 25 and older). By comparing performances for people of different ages, Arthur and Rahe determined that in four free-style events the decline in swim performances over 30 years was nearly identical: approximately 22%. The average falloff in performances came to 0.8% per year. The one event with the most pronounced decline was the butterfly. The investigators theorized that the strength required to swim that stroke caused the greater slowdown. Women declined by 20-50% more than men swimmers, possibly because fewer women competed as Masters.

What was the reason for the general decline? At the end of their study Arthur and Rahe decided that this decline paralleled previous studies by non-athletic researchers on the decline of pulmonary function (the ability of the body to utilize oxygen).

They wrote, "The effects of aging on two measures of a man's pulmonary performance have been shown to approximate a decrement of 1% per year during middle age. (See Table A: Oxygen and Aging.) Hence, the same estimate derived from the men's record Masters swim times suggests a 'biological constant'—perhaps the total of the aging process. If muscle strength alone determined swim performance, the falloff over the 30 years under study should have been curvilinear and closer to a mean estimate of 0.33% per year. Thus, one might presume that it is the decrease in

Table A: Oxygen and Aging

In a study entitled "Age and Aerobic Capacity of Urban Midwestern Males," J.L. Hodgson of the University of Minnesota measured the maximum oxygen uptake (in milliliters of air divided by body weight per minute) of men he described as "moderately active." These included former athletes or men active by occupation or recreation. It suggests the rate at which our lungs will fail us.

Age	Max.	Age	Max.	Age	Max.
20	52.8	33	47.1	46	41.4
21	52.4	34	46.6	47	40.9
22	51.9	35	46.2	48	40.5
23	51.5	36	45.8	49	40.0
24	51.0	37	45.3	50	39.6
25	50.6	38	44.9	51	39.2
26	50.2	39	44.4	52	38.7
27	49.7	40	44.0	53	38.3
28	49.3	41	43.6	54	37.8
29	48.8	42	43.1	55	37.4
30	48.4	43	42.7	56	37.0
31	48.0	44	42.2	57	36.5
32	47.5	45	41.8	59	35.6

pulmonary function that chiefly influences decrease in man's swim performances over his middle-age years."

Peter Mundle, of Venice, Calif., who edits an annual compilation of track and field records entitled *Age Records* for *Track & Field News*, made a similar study of the decline in performances by athletes aged 40-60 years. He identified a deterioration of basically 0.2 second per 100 meters per year at distances from 100 yards to the mile, and 0.3 second per 100 meters per year from two miles to the marathon. This would mean that a 1500-meter runner would find himself growing slower by three seconds each year.

Ken Young, director of the National Running Data Center in Tucson, Ariz., made a similar study specially for this book on the performance of athletes in the 100 meters, mile and marathon. He showed a rate of decline in the mile (the competitive equivalent of the 1500 meters) somewhat less than that indicated by Mundle. A miler who runs the "magic" time of four minutes at the optimal age for his event of 25 will see his performance deteriorate to 4:07 by age 35, to 4:37 by age 50 and to 6:20 by age 80. A 10-flat 100-meter sprinter will suffer similar declines from 10.5 to 11.6 to 15.9. A marathon runner capable of covering 26 miles 385 yards in 2 1/2 hours will slide from 2:32:10 to 2:53:00 to 4:03:00. Similar declines can be predicted for less gifted athletes who run those events in 11-flat, five minutes and three hours while at their prime.

Young's charts related to these three events are printed later in this chapter. A more complete statistical breakdown on the effects of aging on athletic performance can be found in the tables in Chapter Eight. Older athletes interested in determining how fast they *might* have accomplished a given event, had they performed at the age of *supposed* maximum athletic efficiency, will also find a table of percentages which will enable them to measure the true value of their achievement against athletes of all ages.

Alas, we must use the term "supposed" athletic efficiency, because a statistician is only as good as his statistics. Ken Young derived his tables from current age-group records, which probably are not a measure of the body's true potential by rather of the performance of current athletes. Competition for older track and field athletes and swimmers has only been occurring for a decade.

David H.R. Pain of San Diego started the first all-event Masters track and field meet (for runners 40 and over) in 1968. Ransom Arthur, M.D., also then located in San Diego, began a Masters swim meet (for swimmers 25 and older, in recognition of the fact that world-class swimmers retire sooner than runners) several years later. Many of the competitors in these programs are individuals who have not competed continuously, but rather returned to their youthful sports when competition became available. Thus, the quality of many of the older age-group records is, at best, suspect.

The performances of a few super-athletes in the older age categories such as New Zealand's Jack Foster (2:11:18 in the marathon at age 41) or California's Bill Fitzgerald (1:58.4 in the 880 at age 47) support this contention. As older athletes who never retired appear on the Masters scene, the rate of decline may prove to be much less precipitous than now seems the case.

The aging process does continue at a certain specified rate, but at different rates for different individuals and in a manner that physiologists still do not understand.

"We don't know much about the deterioration of the nervous system," admits Richard J. Jones, M.D., a gerontologist with the American Medical Association. "The ultimate deterioration is senility, and the presumption is that it is due to hardening of the arteries leading to the brain. But many patients develop senility without much hardening of the arteries."

According to *Timiras,* a standard physiology textbook, "Differences in sex, past history, heredity, medical history, etc. make the aging process different for each individual. It is practically impossible to separate age-related cellular changes from pathological cellular changes associated with disease of old age."

Certain changes are more predictable than others. Usually between age 40 and 44, the eyes of most people lose their ability to change the shape of the intraocular lenses (those inside the eye which focus it). The result of this condition is they now must wear bifocals. The reason for this loss of ability is that the cornea is made up of collagen, which becomes rigid as one gets older. The number of optic nerves serving vision decreases. A person competing in a sport requiring hand-eye coordination (baseball,

Table B: Running Slowdown Rates

100 METERS

Optimal Age (22)	10.0	11.0
30	10.2	11.2
35	10.5	11.5
40	10.8	11.9
45	11.2	12.3
50	11.6	12.8
55	12.2	13.4
60	12.9	14.2
65	13.6	15.0
70	14.3	15.8
75	15.1	16.6
80	15.9	17.4

MILE

Optimal Age (25)	4:00	5:00
30	4:03	5:03
35	4:07	5:09
40	4:15	5:19
45	4:25	5:33
50	4:37	5:46
55	4:52	6:04
60	5:07	6:24
65	5:25	6:46
70	5:43	7:08
75	6:01	7:32
80	6:20	7:55

	MARATHON	
Optimal Age (29)	**2:30:00**	**3:00:00**
30	2:30:09	3:00:11
35	2:32:10	3:02:50
40	2:37:10	3:09:20
45	2:44:20	3:18:20
50	2:53:00	3:29:20
55	3:02:45	3:42:00
60	3:13:30	3:55:45
65	3:25:10	4:10:30
70	3:37:20	4:26:15
75	3:50:00	4:42:30
80	4:03:10	4:59:20

tennis) may find himself unable to compete equally with other athletes despite the condition of the rest of his body.

Similarly, other parts of the body deteriorate. The number of olfactory nerve fibers (which regulate the sense of smell) decline steadily until at age 90 a person has 25% of those he had at birth. Lean body mass (the skeletal muscles and all other cellular tissues) decrease steadily, so that by extreme old age a person retains only two-thirds the amount found in young adults. At the same time, body weight increases due to stored fat and increased body water in excess of the loss of lean body mass.

The loss of voluntary muscle tissue mass, however, results as much from the lack of exercise as the loss of muscle fibers. Collagen, one of the essential fibrous proteins mentioned earlier in connection with the eye, also is found in the skin, bones and tendons. At an early age, much of a person's collagen is soluble. But as he ages, more and more of it becomes insoluble, causing a decreased permeability of the tissues to dissolved nutrients, hormones and antibodies.

Another essential to the body is elastin, a molecule responsible for the elasticity of the blood vessel walls. With age, there is a loss of elasticity, presumably because of fragmentation of the elastin molecule. Because of these factors, the body gets stiffer as it gets older.

The bones of the body also suffer a decline. Osteoarthritis often begins in the fourth decade of a person's life. The bones develop osteoporosis, losing calcium and becoming more opaque. Bones in most people become thin in their 50s and 60s. By their 70s, they will break easily. Fractures occur more often to older people, with women (whose troubles begin following menopause) having more problems than men. Physiologists do not know why.

Yet part of the deterioration of the human body—in fact, *much* of it—may be due less to the so-called "aging process," which theoretically affects every human being at a statistically predictable rate, than it is due to the fact that most people lose their interest in exercise and fitness once they leave their teens. Athletes have stronger bones than sedentary individuals, but are they successful athletes because of stronger bones (and bodies) or do they develop stronger bones (and bodies) because they become athletes?

No one knows for sure, but many physicians suspect that the latter is more true than the former. According to Dr. Philip Spiegel of the University of Chicago, "The more active one is, the less likely one's bones will get thin, because bones respond to stress by getting thicker."

Dr. Richard J. Jones of the American Medical Association adds, "Physical activity, and straining and tugging on bones, helps develop them no matter what the person's age. When you flex your muscles, your bones become harder."

Dr. Jones suggests another theory of aging: "As we go through life, we pick up a series of insults: infarctions, abscesses, torn muscles, broken bones, calcium deposits. A heart attack leaves a scar on the heart. A stroke does the same on the brain. A person might lose an arm or a leg. Certain materials in the cells don't get digested or excreted. The liver cells may deteriorate and not be able to cope with the body wastes. The cells carry around an excess burden of material which they cannot digest or excrete, and this affects the digestive functions of the cells. Over the years, all of these accidents add up until the point where a person no longer can carry on."

Perhaps the single most debilitating "insult" to the body in 20th century America is atherosclerosis, heart disease characterized by fatty deposits (cholesterol and other complex substances) in the arteries that lead to the heart. These deposits eventually accumulate in the arteries, like rust in a pipe, until the passage of blood to the heart or brain is blocked. The result in the first instance is a heart attack, in the second a stroke.

According to Richard J. Jones, M.D., "Probably the most important part of of the body is the arteries. A man over 40 would do best to preserve his arteries above all else, because that is the canal that keeps blood flowing to the heart and brain."

In past years, scientists used to believe that atherosclerosis was not only inevitable, but also irreversible. But recent evidence, according to Dr. Jones, suggests that the development of plaque in the arteries, at least in the early stages, not only can be halted but may be reversed. If a person changes his diet or exercises sufficiently to burn up excessive fats in the blood stream, the cells on the artery walls may diminish in both size and number.

"There is probably a point beyond which the process does not reverse," admits Dr. Jones, "such as if there is too much scar tissue. But the important point is that man may be more in control of his destiny than he thinks."

And athletes may find that with proper utilization of their resources, they are less likely to decline than they, or physiologists, or statisticians, think. Man may not prove himself immortal, but he may find himself capable of living not only a longer but a fuller life than he now believes possible.

During the summer of 1976, a team of educators from the Department of Heath, Education and Welfare appeared at a school district south of Chicago for which I do work in a consulting capacity. It was a preliminary stage of a program to educate teachers in preventive health. It was hoped the teachers then would pass the message on to their pupils. When Roy Davis, director of HEW's Community Program Development Division, visited the school I had an opportunity to talk with him about man's capacity to affect his own health.

Davis told me, "We are now getting to the point where everybody has to decide if they are going to drink and how much, what they are going to eat and how much, and if they are going to exercise and how much, if they are going to use the health care system or whether they will avoid care."

Davis paused as though admitting that the answers to those questions would prove unsatisfactory. He confirmed it with his next statement: "Unfortunately, people are not always making the best decisions for themselves."

But human beings, particularly those over 40, can greatly improve their physical fitness if only they will try to do so.

2

A Disneyland for Joggers

Driving in my rental car up the driveway of the fashionable club with its handsome Colonial-style buildings on the north side of Dallas, Texas, I slowed before a traffic sign. It signified a pedestrian crossing—visually, not with words; the kind of sign you see more frequently in Europe. Instead of the silhouette of a person walking, however, it showed a person *running*. It was the driveway of Dr. Kenneth H. Cooper's Aerobics Center where running—or, perhaps more precisely, jogging—is very much the favored activity.

Dr. Cooper, a former space scientist, in 1968 authored the book *Aerobics*, which has sold nearly eight million copies in various editions and in 19 different languages. After leaving the Air Force, he founded his Center in suburban Dallas as a place where he could: (a) practice medicine; (b) supervise fitness research; (c) provide an athletic opportunity for men and women who were beyond what many Americans considered the athletic age, and (d) do some jogging himself. It is the dream of many runners to own their own track, and Dr. Cooper fulfilled that dream.

The Aerobics Center might be described as a "Disneyland for joggers." Its neatly landscaped grounds contain a soft-surfaced half-mile jogging path that winds beneath groves of trees and around a pond occupied by ducks and geese. Branching off that half-mile path is another quarter-mile loop. The setting has the delicacy of a Japanese garden. It is rare to visit the Aerobics Center at any time between 6 a.m. and 10 p.m. Mondays through Saturdays and not see at least several people jogging around these paths. In peak hours—in the morning before members go to downtown jobs or in the evening after work—Aerobics Center paths reverberate to the rhythm of hundreds of rubberized shoes.

But the Aerobics Center includes more than jogging on its daily schedule. The sprawling complex also includes a gymnasium for basketball, volleyball and exercise classes. Around the gym floor is an indoor track (24 laps to the mile) with electronic pacer lights set in the floor and adjustable to any speed (such as a 12-minute-per-mile pace for a man told to jog at that speed while recovering from a heart attack). On a balcony above are exercise bikes and a Universal Gym for weight lifting activities.

Outside is a 25-yard heated pool. Its lanes can be reserved by the hour for distance swimming, just as one might reserve a racquetball court. Two such courts are at the other end of the building. Behind the parking lot (which contains more Cadillacs than Volkswagens) are four lighted tennis courts.

Indeed, the Aerobics Center contains everything you might expect in a fashionable country club, *except* a bar and a golf course. The Center does have a non-alcoholic snack bar, where executives can grab a quick breakfast following a morning jog and before going to work, but meals there favor nutrition over empty calories. The specialty of the day is a mammoth pineapple, hollowed out and filled with raspberries, strawberries, melons and assorted other fruits. For a drink along with this main course: apple cider. For dessert: an oatmeal cookie. The Aerobics Center snack bar, in fact, may be the only restaurant in Dallas worthy of four stars in, if not the *Michelin Guide Book*, then the *Joggers' Guide*.

The man who founded Aerobics, Kenneth H. Cooper, M.D., M.P.H., sits in his paneled office sipping a glass of Gatorade (his strongest drink) to soothe a throat sore from too many speeches in too few days. He is wearing the standard, knee-length, white physician's jacket. He leans back in his swivel chair and crosses his legs. He is a thin, tall, ascetic-appearing man who, because he promotes physical fitness with almost evangelical fervor, has been likened to an athletic Messiah.

Filling the shelves behind Dr. Cooper are copies of the foreign editions of his *Aerobics* books, which have been translated into 19 languages, including Russian. An edition in that country published in the summer of 1976 sold out 75,000 copies in two weeks.

Ken Cooper has written three books. In addition to his 1968 *Aerobics*, he wrote *The New Aerobics* (1970) and *Aerobics for Women* (1972), written with his wife Millie. All were published in paperback so they are easily available to more people. The books offer plain, simple advice on how first to get in shape, then although they are available. He claims that he wants them in paperback so they are more easily available to more people. The books offer plain, simple adivce on how first to get in shape then how to stay in shape. Whenever anyone who has never run before approaches me asking how they can enter the Boston Marathon, I always tell him, "Go read *Aerobics* first."

Although Dr. Cooper makes no pretense of producing literature, he is probably better known in some foreign countries than probably better known in some foreign countries than recent Nobel Prize author Saul Bellow, particularly in Brazil where Dr. Cooper once spoke before 240,000 people in a stadium during a Billy Graham evangelistic crusade. Dr. Cooper gave a 10-minute testimony on the interrelationship between spiritual and physical fitness. A photograph on the wall autographed by Billy Graham and showing the packed stadium commemorates that event on Oct. 6, 1974, and Dr. Cooper called my attention to it soon after I entered his office.

In Brazil, the Portugese-speaking population had difficulty pronouncing the word "Aerobics," so when the city of Rio de Janeiro established a jogging path with stops for exercises in a public park, they named it a "Cooper Course."

Dr. Cooper smiles as he relates the incident, aware of the touch of immortality it provides him while at the same time providing an extension, perhaps, on the *mortality* of the residents of Rio. He quotes Carleton Chapman, M.D., former president of the American Heart Association, who once stated that the use of exercise in preventing heart disease was in a state of transition from "unfounded faddism to scientific legitimacy."

Dr. Cooper claims, "I've spent my professional life trying to bridge that gap."

Perhaps the single contribution that Ken Cooper made in improving the fitness of millions throughout the world is that he was the man who uncovered an easily understood method of quantifying exercise. Others had attempted to quantify exercise before, but none had done it quite so well. His best-selling book, *Aerobics*, contains a series of charts giving relative point values to different types of exercise.

For example, a mile jogged in 10 minutes is worth four points. Five miles of bicycle riding in 20 minutes equals five points. A four-mile walk in one hour earns seven points. If at the end of each week, an individual interested in proving his or her physical fitness accumulates 30-34 points (Dr. Cooper's benchmark of fitness), that person can significantly lower five of the 10 risk factors causing coronary heart attacks.* Before Dr. Cooper appeared, most physicians assumed exercise benefited their patients; he showed them how much.

At the Aerobics Center in Dallas, members record their daily exercise by means of a keyboard at the desk outside the locker room hooked into a computer. They can determine, within seconds, the value of their just-completed exercise to one-hundredth of a point. At various intervals, they can discover how many points they have earned per week, how many miles run, how many yards swum, how many hours of racquetball played (although the computer is not programmed to record scores or won-lost records). If they so desire, they can obtain a computer feedback of what they have accomplished in the area of exercise fitness.

This computer feedback becomes part of a reward system,

---

* The five risk factors lowered are: (1) cholesterol; (2) glucose; (3) triglycerides; (4) body weight and body fat, and (5) systolic and diastolic blood pressure.

points instead of medals or trophies. It might be compared to a mouse in a psychologist's experiment who learns he will be rewarded if he nudges one lever and shocked if he nudges another. The shock, for people who do not use the system, could be a heart attack.

Although a system for quantifying physical exercise that utilizes a computer to determine values to the one-hundredth percentile seems complex and extreme, the beauty of Dr. Cooper's system—and the reason for its popularity—is its basic simplicity. A person who buys one of his books can use the charts contained therein to determine, without a computer and in a matter of seconds, the number of points earned for most basic exercises.

As long as Ken Cooper does have access to a computer, however, he uses it to also keep precise exercise records on himself as well as on his patients. He pulls a printout sheet from his desk drawer and informs me that, since 1960, he has run 15,816 miles. While the sum might seem monumental to a sendentary individual, it actually is paltry by Olympian standards. (Frank Shorter, the Olympic gold and silver medalist in the marathon, averages 140 miles a week in training and would cover that much mileage in little over two years' time.) A typical workout for Ken Cooper is a gentle three-mile jog around the paths at his Aerobics Center. He preaches temperance in fitness.

"Our most popular program," says Dr. Cooper, "and the one I recommend most, is only two miles in 20 minutes four times a week. That's a very reasonable workout, and the vast majority of American people can work up to that, even until 50 or 60 years of age."

Born in Oklahoma City on March 4, 1931, Kenneth H. Cooper in 1949 made all-state in basketball and won the state mile championship, running 4:30.8. While attending the University of Oklahoma, he ran on several winning two-mile and four-mile relay teams at the Texas and Drake Relays.

Many physicians find it difficult to maintain a program of physical fitness while facing the grind of medical school and residency requirements. Dr. Cooper, however, never lost his interest in fitness. In the early 1960s, while taking post-graduate work at the Harvard School of Public Health, he decided to enter the Boston Marathon, which despite its world-wide reputation seldom, at this time, attracted more than a few hundred entrants. With the possible exception of the handful of top athletes up front, anyone who entered the race was considered by the general public to be some kind of nut.

"I ran the Boston Marathon twice," admits Dr. Cooper, who hardly fits the general public's image. "The first time was in 1962, and I was the last official finisher. I ran the distance in 3:54 and came in 101st place. My name was the last one in the newspaper, and the only reason it was recorded was because my wife insisted the judges stay until I got in. They were ready to leave at 3 1/2 hours."

He improved his time by nearly 40 minutes in 1963 but only improved his place by two positions. He finished 99th. More and better runners entered that year's event; the interest in long-distance running already had begun. *Sports Illustrated* published an article on marathoning, focused on Boston and entitled "On the Run from Dogs and People" in 1963.* The list of entrants doubled the following year, proving the power of the press. Today, officials of the Boston Marathon limit entrants to those capable of finishing under three hours (3 1/2 hours for women and runners 40 and older), yet roughly 2,000 hopefuls still appear. Additional thousands compete in the nearly 200 other marathons across the United States, many of them having taken their first running step after reading *Aerobics*.

But this all happened later. After completing his studies at Harvard, Dr. Cooper was assigned by the Air Force to its Manned Orbiting Laboratory program near San Antonio, Tex. It was a heady time for a young physician: to be connected, even tangentially, to a project which would result in placing man on the moon. The space program involved not merely constructing a powerful enough rocket to launch man into space and designing the complicated computerized guidance systems to make millisecond course corrections. Another important factor was to see that the astronauts were conditioned to withstand the tremendous physical demands on their bodies, which included forces many times the pull of gravity during launch and the deteriorating

---

* Written by Hal Higdon. That was also the name of a book by him on long distance running published by Regnery in 1969.

effects of weightlessness in deep space.

This latter problem was particularly a concern for those connected with the Manned Orbiting Laboratory project, to which Dr. Cooper was assigned, because of the long periods to be spent in space. The astronauts were superb physical specimens with extremely high motivation. But what exercises were best for them both to prepare for and during weightlessness? And how much exercise? Those were some of the questions that Dr. Cooper sought to answer through biomedical research.

One day in 1966, Kevin Brown, a *Popular Mechanics* editor doing an article on the astronauts, visited Lackland Air Force Base in San Antonio where Dr. Cooper was stationed. He spent one entire week moving from office to office, talking to one scientist after another, usually for an hour. Brown became particularly fascinated by what he learned in the time spent in Dr. Cooper's office.

"Can I come back and talk to you later?" asked Brown before moving on to his next appointment.

Dr. Cooper said yes, and the two later collaborated on an article under Dr. Cooper's byline for *Family Weekly*, a Sunday supplement distributed mostly with small city newspapers. Following publication of the article, the two produced *Aerobics*, also under Dr. Cooper's byline, and it became a best-selling paperback not because it told people that they could live longer by physical exercise, but because it showed them *how*.

Kevin Brown is not associated with the Aerobics Center (and did not participate in the writing of Dr. Cooper's other two books), but he continues to jog regularly: up to five miles a workout, three or four workouts a week, for a total of 10 miles weekly.

Dr. Cooper had very definite ideas as to what it took to achieve total physical fitness, and it was not the easy five or 10 minutes a day that later get-fit-quick proponents suggested. In that first edition of *Aerobics*, he wrote, "After four years of searching for it, I can lay down two basic principles. If your program is limited to 12-20 minutes a day of activity, the exercise must be vigorous enough to produce a sustained heart rate of 150 beats per minute or more. If the exercise is not vigorous enough to produce a sustained heart rate of 150 beats per minute, but is still demanding oxygen, the exercise must be continued longer than 20 minutes, the total period of time depending on the oxygen consumed."*

The title of Dr. Cooper's book related to oxygen use. Aerobic means "able to live or grow only where free oxygen is present." Anaerobic means "able to live or grow where there is no free oxygen." Jogging is an aerobic activity, because it takes place over a relatively long period of time, meaning the body must continuously replenish its oxygen supplies to keep moving. Sprinting, on the other hand, is an anaerobic activity, because it is completed so fast that the body can use the oxygen already within its system. Sprinters usually finish gasping for breath; joggers do not.

The publication *Aerobics*, and its subsequent popularity, helped raise the health consciousness of many Americans, teaching them to balance their exercise accounts as they might their bank accounts. In the early 1960s, the only people seen running in public were a few dedicated long-distance runners, happy in their supposed loneliness, many of them young and with Olympic ambitions. They were so rare that bystanders snickered at them, teenagers in cars yelled insults at them, and dogs chased and bit them. Today, the number of people running in public has escalated to the point where the runner or jogger no longer is a novelty, either on the YMCA track or running along a sidewalk in the fanciest subdivision. No longer the property of the young, running/jogging has been taken over by men and women into their 60s and 70s. Runners/joggers have become part of the scenery. Bystanders no longer snicker, teenagers are into other activities, and even dogs have lost interest and gone back to chasing cars.

In 1974, the President's Council on Physical Fitness and Sports released a survey on adult exercise habits. The vast majority of regular exercisers claimed walking as that activity. The study indicated, however, that six million jogged. It did not say how often, but just said they jogged, which could include running in place in their living room while watching "Kojak."

---

* Dr. Cooper's rule is probably workable for the average human being, but not for trained distance runners who have much lower heartbeats. For example, my maximum heartbeat (tested on one of Dr. Cooper's own treadmills; see Chapter 15) is 160 beats per minute. An equivalent sustained exercise level for me would be 120, instead of 150, beats per minute.

Dr. Cooper suggests the figure should be higher: "There were 10,000 people competing in marathons last year," he states, "and that's just the tip of the iceberg. If you have that many people actually competing in marathons, what's the volume like down at the bottom? I think 10 million is a realistic guess."

Perhaps an even more significant statistic is that deaths from heart attacks had been increasing steadily in the United States since 1940, but in 1968 (the year of publication of *Aerobics*), the curve turned downward for the first time. The percentage of deaths from heart attacks decreased nearly 13% in the following eight years. The number, however, still is frightening: more than 600,000 a year.

It would be wrong to claim a direct cause and effect relationship between Dr. Cooper's book and the decrease in heart attack deaths. Dr. Cooper shuns credit for either the jogging explosion or the decline in heart attack deaths but points to the latter when rebutting critics who suggest the former is dangerous.

"Obviously people aren't dying by the hundreds from jogging, or that would be reflected in the statistics," he says.

One critic of Dr. Cooper's exercise theories (Dr. Meyer Friedman, co-author of *Type A Behavior and Your Heart*) predicted one problem requiring resuscitation for every 1000 miles jogged, one death per 10,000 miles. Members of the Aerobics Center in Dallas logged their millionth mile during the summer of 1976 with no deaths and only one case requiring resuscitation.

One master sergeant did die of a heart attack while participating in Dr. Cooper's Air Force program. The sergeant, 51 years old, had three-vessel heart disease. He was stricken 45 minutes after running a 1.5-mile field test and died 11 days later, sending shock waves through Cooper's staff, who feared that adverse reaction would cause the program's cancellation. But in the next six months, 15,000 subjects had no further heart attacks or deaths.

"Just from statistics alone," says Dr. Cooper, "we could have predicted at last three heart attacks and at least one death among this large group of men. At these same five bases, there were 12,000 men who weren't on the exercise program. They sat back and laughed at their buddies. During this period, their group had nine heart attacks and two deaths. So if you ask me how many people have been killed by Aerobics, I'll ask you how many people wouldn't be here today if they hadn't exercised?

"You hear of isolated cases because they're newsworthy," continues Dr. Cooper. "People die while jogging, just like they die playing golf, walking down the street or sleeping in bed. You have 600,000 people a year dying of heart attacks, so obviously a lot of people could be doing a lot of things. I keep telling my audiences that, unfortunately, jogging does not carry with it immortality. You might die jogging, but you have to keep things within perspective."

Nevertheless, he cautions persons attempting any physical exercise program that they should obtain a complete physical examination (preferably including a stress test) to rule out the possibility of any abnormal physical problems that might rule out exercise. Such an examination is a requirement for anyone becoming a member of the Aerobics Center.

He reacts strongly to the publication of recent articles, particularly one in the *New York Times*, suggesting that annual physical examinations were of little value.*

"Many health exams are worthless," he concedes, "but the type of comprehensive complete examination we do here is extremely valuable. The article criticizing exams failed to mention the use of stress tests on treadmills. Twelve per cent of the patients that come to our clinic have abnormal stress tests. Twelve per cent of 10,000 patients is a lot of patients. They have heart disease, and it never was diagnosed before."

"If we can pick out this problem early and help the patient change the risk factors, and motivate him to exercise, we may save his life. We have people who move from a high coronary risk factor to a low coronary risk factor in a period as short as six months. There are many things you can do once you have diagnosed problems, but most people in this country are not preventive-oriented.

"There was another article in the *New York Times* (Dec. 1, 1975) by Ashley Montague, entitled 'Rehumanizing Medicine,' and he said that for too many years preventive medicine has been

---

* "The Case Against Regular Physicals," by Richard Spark, M.D., *The New York Times Magazine*, July 25, 1976. See Chapter 15 of this book for a discussion on the subject.

the cinderella of the medical specialties. They talk about it, but they don't do it.

"He claimed there were two reasons. Number one, too many of us never see a doctor except when we're sick, and we associate physicians with sickness, not with health. We are going to have to resort back to the concepts of ancient China where they paid their physicians when they were healthy. They didn't pay their physicians when they were sick.

"The second thing he said is that physicians in this country are not trained in preventive medicine and they have little interest in it. People have the idea that there is no profit in health, and certainly there is not as much profit in this organization as you would have in a center doing open heart surgery. But look at the escalating cost of medical care in this country: $150 billion predicted for 1977. That compares with $12 billion in 1950, $70 billion in 1970, $118 billion in 1975. We've doubled the cost of medical care in this country in six years. We've made tremendous advances in medicine, but they're all very expensive. Yet there is little profit thus far in preventive medicine."

Seeing the value of exercise through his studies, Dr. Cooper, in 1968, attempting to convince the Air Force to fund a special facility for fitness. When the government denied his request, he decided to resign his commission as lieutenant colonel and obtain private financing for a civilian facility. His Aerobics Center, costing $2 million to construct, now has 1350 members, one-third of them women. Most female members are housewives who use the facilities during the day. Male members appear most often in the hours before and after work, and on weekends.

Utilization of the Center is extremely high: 75% of the members appear at least once a week, compared to a utilization rate of 40% for a standard health club. On any given day, 50% of the members will work out at the facilities, which are closed only on Sundays, in keeping with Dr. Cooper's religious beliefs. Fifty communities have approached him with the idea of organizing Aerobics Centers elsewhere, but he has resisted the temptation to become the McDonald's of Fitness.

"The average age of our member is 45," explains Bill Grantham, physical director of the Aerobics Center in Dallas. "He is typically a senior executive for whom money is no particular problem, but he now finds that his health has begun to slide on him, and *that* is very important to him. He will spend almost any amount of money to get his health back: to get weight off, to lower his blood pressure, to drop that cholesterol or triglyceride reading or whatever. He is an individual smart enough to know that his health relates to his ability to accomplish things, so the cost of health is relatively unimportant."

The price of health, if that means joining the Aerobics Center, is not low. Membership in the Center costs $475 annually, probably less than most country clubs but more than membership in the typical YMCA. Considering that a stay in the average American hospital cost $175 a day in 1976, it still may be a bargain. It is worth noting that at no place in the Aerobics Center can one lounge, alcoholic drink in hand, and watch *others* exercise.

A physician is present on the facilities from opening at 6 o'clock in the morning to closing at 10 at night, but rarely is one called upon for emergency care. The only two exceptions were one person who had an epiletic seizure and another individual who suffered a cardiac arrythmia. The latter was a visitor to the Center who, without sufficient preparation, entered the Tyler Cup, a fitness-oriented track meet for executives that the Center sponsors each year. He later joined the Center, and after a year and a half continues to exercise without further problems.

Most of their work day, the five physicians (including Dr. Cooper himself) connected with what is referred to as the Cooper Clinic busy themselves giving thorough, exercise-oriented physical examinations and supervising a load of 10,000 patients who, after being examined, follow regular exercise programs planned for them. The practice has a return rate of 65-70%. The waiting list for those wanting initial physical examinations at the Cooper Clinic is six months long, with individuals obtaining appointments usually only if someone else cancels. The only speedy way to obtain such a physical examination is to become a member of the Aerobics Center, for which a complete checkup, including stress test, replaces the standard initiation rites of most other clubs.

A third phase of the program is research on exercise fitness which continues at a separate facility nearby, under the supervision of physiologist Michael Pollock who tests overweight executives as well as world-class athletes like Frank Shorter or the late Steve Prefontaine. Equipment in this test facility includes a submersion tank by which a test subject is weighed while totally immersed in water so that the percentage of body fat can be precisely determined. To be judged as not overweight, a man should have a body fat reading below 19%, women below 22%. Most competitive long-distance runners have body fat percentages below 10%; most champions around 5%.

Test subjects also run on treadmills, their every heartbeat monitored by electrocardiograms, their oxygen consumption measured by a tube covering their mouths and connected to a collecting device. By raising the incline of the treadmill or increasing its speed, Center researchers can simulate in the laboratory the stress undergone by an athlete running a four-minute mile or a full-distance marathon of 26 miles 385 yards.

The three basic activities of the Aerobics Center—exercise, examination and research—spin merrily along without Dr. Cooper's constant presence, a necessity because of his frequent absences from Dallas. He gives between 75 and 125 lectures ("presentations," he calls them) a year, many of them before medical and dental groups. ("The dentists were the first ones to discover me," he says. "They stand in place at their jobs all day and get very little exercise.")

Dr. Cooper's presentations vary from 30 minutes after a luncheon to a six-hour session. He claims to have enough material so he can talk for 12 hours without duplicating what he says. Frequently, he leaves Dallas at 6 a.m., travels more than 1000 miles to a meeting, speaks for hours, then returns home by midnight. Often, he will be gone for a week, spending each day in a different city.

"It is very demanding," he admits. "If you do a couple of six-hour presentations back to back in two cities, you are shot."

He refuses as many speaking engagements as he accepts, avoiding most typical luncheon groups who might think of him only as entertainment, and concentrates on groups whose members might become disciples to spread his word to others. He speaks only nine months of the year, avoiding engagements either in December or in July and August, to permit him more time with his family.

He is a spellbinding speaker, capable of totally captivating an audience. "You almost have to become an actor," he suggests, "to create the same enthusiasm in presenting material you know like the back of your hand. But audiences turn me on. Like a group up in Hamilton, Ontario, the other night. There were about 250 people, and when I asked for a show of hands as to how many jogged, about 90% raised their hands. That's when I know I have a captive audience."

Dr. Cooper also remembers warmly an appearance before a group of physicians with the Hospital Corporation of America, a privately run chain of hospitals. "That was the only group that gave me a standing ovation *before* I walked up to the platform," he recalls, a trace of emotion crossing his usually stoic features.

The hospital chain had approached Dr. Cooper with the idea of their sponsoring a fitness relay for their physicians, each participant jogging two miles. The person in charge of the event wondered how many participants to expect at such an event? Dr. Cooper asked how many hospitals were in their chain, and when the person said 76, he estimated that 25 or 30 physicians might participate. As it turned out, 208 physicians representing 70% of the hospitals in the chain participated, the fastest being a 29-year-old doctor from Florida who covered the two-mile distance in 9:59.

"These were my men," says Dr. Cooper with a smile.

"Anyone capable of running two miles at that speed—or even at a speed several minutes slower—would be classified by Dr. Cooper as being in "excellent" shape. In *Aerobics*, he shows how people (those who have been exercising fairly regularly) can test themselves by determining how far they can go—walking, jogging or any combination of both—in 12 minutes. He thus rates them in five categories of fitness, as follows:

If You Cover . . .	You Are In Fitness Category . . .
less than 1.0 mile	I — Very Poor
1.0 to 1.24 miles	II — Poor
1.25 to 1.49 miles	III — Fair
1.50 to 1.74 miles	IV — Good
1.75 miles or more	V — Excellent

For anyone over 35 years of age who had not been exercising regularly, he recommended beginning with a preliminary conditioning program of walking, swimming, cycling, running or several other sports to get in condition to take the test. For example, the following chart for a 40-year-old swimmer was presented in *The New Aerobics:**

Week	Distance (yards)	Time (min.)	Frequency Wk.	Points/Wk.
1	100	2:30	5	4
2	150	3:15	5	5
3	175	4:00	5	6
4	200	4:30	5	7½
5	200	4:15	5	7½
6	250	5:30	5	10

Conditioning programs for different activities and age categories showed a similar easy progression. A person who built himself up to this minimal level of fitness then was encouraged to take the 12-minute test.

Dr. Cooper explains the significance of test results: "We have excellent correlations between coronary risk factors and points. We know the people who reach the 'Good' category of fitness have significant differences in coronary risk factors compared to those in the 'Fair' to 'Very Poor' categories."

Dr. Cooper's book showed how individuals might improve themselves from "Very Poor" to "Poor" and from "Poor" to "Fair," and beyond, by a systematized schedule of exercise. Each sport engaged in at a certain level of activity produced a certain number of points. For example, a mile run earned an individual the following points, depending on the time in which it was run:

Time	Points
14:29-12:00	2
11:59-10:00	3
9:59-8:00	4
7:59-6:30	5
under 6:30	6

* Using the overhand crawl; breaststroke is less demanding and so is backstroke; butterfly is considerably more demanding.

Similar points could be earned by cycling, for example, six miles at different speeds:

Time	Points
36:00 or longer	1
35:59-24:00	3
23:59-18:00	6
under 18:00	9

A person engaging in swimming, walking, stationery running, handball, squash or basketball also earned points depending on duration or speed. Dr. Cooper even could show you the relative value of skiing and rope skipping. He recommended obtaining between 30 and 34 points in a week, regardless of the type of activity.

With *The New Aerobics*, in 1970, he offered a different scale of exercises for different ages, not available in his first book. *Aerobics for Women*, in 1972, offered charts for women. But the goal was always 30 to 34 points.

Dr. Cooper states, "I can sit right here and tell you that if you get 34 points a week, you can reduce five of the 10 coronary risk factors. There will be a significant difference between your health and the health of those walking around who get less. I don't care if you get your points walking, running, cycling, swimming or what; you can improve your health. Going beyond that, as most competitive athletes do, does not seem to make much difference. A person who earns 50 points a week doesn't improve his statistical chances over the person earning 30 to 34, although if he enjoys doing it, fine.

"We are evaluating exercise in a very sophisticated manner, like you would take a new antibiotic and study its effect. Overdoses can kill people. Underdoses are not effective. So what is the dose most effective in reversing coronary infarctions? No one used exercise this way because they said you couldn't quantify it. But now we have terms by which we can quantify fitness.

"Physicians in this country know nothing about good health, and particularly they know very little about exercise physiology. But our studies show that it is possible for a person to grow healthier as he grows older and not necessarily the reverse."

He continues, "There was an excellent article published not

long ago in the *American Geriatrics Society Journal* by Alton Ochfner from New Orleans, talking about aging. He said that three things accelerate the aging process, in this priority: (1) smoking; (2) inactivity, and (3) obesity. I couldn't agree with him more. I feel that by controlling these three things you can remarkably slow down the aging process.

"I firmly believe that when a man dies, he dies not so much of the diseases he has as he dies of what happened his entire life. We do not die as much as we kill ourselves. The major cause of death in men 35 to 54 years of age are all to some extent preventable: heart disease, lung cancer, automobile accidents, cirrhosis of the liver and stroke."

Dr. Cooper finished ticking these causes off on his fingers and paused to let the effect of his words soak in. We had been talking for nearly an hour, but his previously hoarse voice seemed, if anything, to be getting stronger. He had another patient coming in, the chairman of a large corporation, a 56-year-old man, an individual in exceptional shape. Dr. Cooper said the man's exercise program had become one of the most important parts of his life for the last six years.

Dr. Cooper finished the point about the way in which man usually died by asking a rhetorical question: "How many of these are acts of God and how many of these are acts of men?"

He smiled again, confident that the gap between unfounded faddism and scientific legitimacy was being bridged.

Following my inteview with Dr. Cooper, I went to the carpeted men's dressing room of the Aerobics Center and changed into shorts, T-shirt and running shoes. It was important to listen to what he said, but I also wanted to experience what he believed. The afternoon had grown late now, and the number of joggers using the half-mile jogging path on the Center's landscaped grounds had increased. I stood and watched for a while as the stream of joggers flowed past at a steady, gentle pace. They wore plain, functional, white T-shirts, not the luridly designed shirts with race names like "Blueberry Stomp" and "4th Annual Fell Distance Run" you see when you are around competitive runners.

A statuesque blonde passed at an easy stroll. When I first saw her coming, I thought she was in her early 30s. But as she got closer, I realized she was at least one generation older. Mounted near the entrance to the gym was a large clock so joggers could time themselves. Some glanced at it as they passed; others did not. A man with radio earphones on his head stood near me, adjusting them, ready to run to a different beat. Several others were doing stretching exercises preceding their workout, always a good idea. A pick-up basketball game was going on behind me in the gymnasium. I heard a splash as someone plunged into the pool nearby.

I moved onto the path and began to run, slow at first, near the same pace as those on the path around me. But I am a trained runner, used to workouts of five, 10, 15 miles and more. As I warmed up, I felt the urge to exert myself. I began to move faster, not from a desire to defeat those around me, but because it feels good to run fast. It is a feeling that not all people, who in the interests of physical fitness begin jogging programs, easily achieve. Failure to achieve that feeling—what Dr. Cooper might refer to as the "training effect," and what others call "second wind"—is what defeats many embryo joggers who do not stay at it long enough.

Soon, I was moving at a pace that would take me through four miles in 26:50—not fast for a competitive runner, but faster than those around me. My strides lengthened. I felt myself floating. I leaned into the turns, cutting close to the grass on the inside, hitting the apex like a sports car driver at Watkins Glen, allowing momentum to swing me wide on the outside then dive toward the inside again on the next twist of the path in the other direction: back and forth, left, right, left. It is hard to understand the exhilaration that comes from running free unless you experience it yourself.

After dodging onto the grass to pass one group, I overheard someone say, "There he goes!" Did they resent my presence? Was I invading their turf? Was I as separated from them as they from those whose only exercise was ripping pull-taps off beer cans while watching TV? No matter; I felt a kinship for those slower runners around me whose goals were tied up in fitness and personal well-being rather than in gold medals won at some athletic contest.

I slowed my pace and started to walk. It was dark now and somewhat cooler. The globes lining the path had come on, illuminating the setting in a subtle, subdued manner. It gave the garden jogging path the air of someplace I might have wanted to walk with a girl friend several decades before. I smelled the scent of something fragrant among the bushes by the pond. The ducks and geese placidly enjoyed this haven of theirs in the middle of the grounds, oblivious to the stream of joggers around them. On the road outside the Aerobics Center, obese Dallas residents drove past on their way home from work, also oblivious to the activity within.

I sat down on the stairs outside the gymnasium, removed my shoes, and went in to shower and then to dress. It was a good way to end the day.

3
The Quest for a Coronary-Prone Characteristic

It can be stated with precise mathematical certainty that the majority of the readers of this book—unless they change their patterns of living—will:

1. Die too soon.
2. Enjoy life too little.

This is the burden carried by the average American.

Consider the statistics: Despite easy access to medical facilities, the American male ranks only 17th in longevity among men of the major nations of the world. American women rank 10th, but their death rate from heart disease is the highest of women from any country and is increasing.

"More than half the deaths in the United States today are caused by cardiovascular ailments," claims Lawrence E. Lamb, M.D. "Worse, these ailments are reaching younger and younger people. For this reason, contrary to the popular misconception, our life expectancy has not improved appreciably in the last two decades despite advances elsewhere in the field of health."

The cause is that Americans have passed into what Kenneth H. Cooper, M.D., describes as "an era of physical passivity."

Consider the results of a study conducted some time ago by Dr. M. Gertler of New York University and famed Boston cardiologist Dr. Paul Dudley White. Researchers studied a total of 490 "medically normal" male employees of a large corporation, charting such factors as body build, height, weight, smoking habits and family history. On the basis of a mathematical formula they had devised earlier, they fed the results of the tests into a computer.

The results were startling. The computer identified 32 employees as being highly coronary prone because of their test scores, and within a space of four years 28 of those 32 people had developed heart disease! Only four of those identified as "coronary prone" remained symptom-free. Of the ones stricken, eight had developed angina pectoris and 20 had suffered heart attacks. Five had died.

Sad as it may seem, many of these heart attacks were probably entirely unnecessary. A significant number of these 28—perhaps as many as half—could have escaped heart disease if they had taken what are now clearly recognized preventive steps. This is true for a large majority of the coronary prone people walking (or more likely riding) the streets today; the people who, in the next five, 10 or 20 years will suffer heart attacks in their 30s, 40s and 50s—in their prime of life.

In the United States, particularly, heart disease continues to be a major problem every year. In 1900, heart disease accounted for only 14% of deaths in the United States. Today, it is responsible for more than half. More than 600,000 Americans die of diseases of the heart and blood vessels every year.

As you may suspect, part of the increase in the importance of heart disease in the 20th century is due to the fact that medical science has over the years eliminated or controlled many of the diseases—smallpox, cholera, diptheria, typhod fever and other infections—that preyed on the young. Unfortunately, this only partially explains the increase in coronary deaths. Coronary heart diseases—smallpox, cholera, diphtheria, typhoid fever and other Morris in England, the late Samual Levine, M.D., of Boston and

Herman K. Hellerstein, M.D., of Cleveland have shown that sons are developing heart attacks earlier in life than their fathers.

Why? Perhaps because as a society we have become soft. We have succumbed to the blandishments of the Good Life. We now ride in automobiles, buses or trains instead of walking or bicycling to work. We jam into elevators instead of climbing stairs. Our work demands less physical activity. On top of it, we eat rich food such as thick, marbled steaks that the average workingman could not afford a generation ago. In every home, the refrigerator bulges with milk and ice cream. We sit before television sets in passive enjoyment of someone else's activity.

We're fatter, too, if we're men. In the last few decades, teenage girls, influenced undoubtedly by Hollywood and fashion magazines, have slimmed their figures by eight pounds, whereas teenage boys have added an average of eight pounds to their frames. Autopsies made on teenagers killed in auto accidents have shown that their arteries had already begun to clog with the fatty substance known as "cholesterol plaques." This substance, had its accumulation not been halted by accidental death, would later have blocked coronary arteries and caused their hearts to stop, or it would have clogged the brain arteries and caused a stroke.

American soldiers killed in Korea were similarly examined. Of these young men, averaging 22 years old, 77% suffered from a signficant amount of heart disease as measured by the condition of their arteries. In contrast, only 5% of Korean soldiers killed in military action suffered from such heart disease.

Numerous studies in past years comparing people in vigorous occupations (such as postmen) vs. sedentary jobs (such as clerks) showed less heart disease among the former. In one classic health study comparing London bus conductors (who had to climb stairs to an upper deck) with their drivers, the drivers came out second best.

Recently, while I was in Gainesville, Fla., speaking at a running clinic, the telephone rang in my hotel room. On the line was Charlie Dorsett, my former top sergeant from when I was stationed with the Seventh Army in Stuttgart, West Germany, in the mid-1950s. Charlie read in the newspaper that I was in town and called to say hello. We had not seen each other in two decades, but I made him promise to stop by the hotel.

Later, when I saw Charlie standing in the lobby, it seemed he had aged very little in 20 years though he was now in his 60s. After retiring from the Army, he went to work for the post office in Indianapolis as a letter-carrier. He delivered mail by foot rather than by the motorized vehicles so popular in many cities. Charlie believed there were certain proprieties you should observe. He never cut across a lawn to shortcut from one door to the other. He used the walks even though many homeowners told him to use their lawns. As a result, he probably walked twice as much as necessary. And as a further result, he remained in excellent physical condition.

After retiring from the post office, Charlie Dorsett moved down to Gainesville, where he found himself gaining weight. In several years, he put on 20 pounds, and he did not like the feeling of being out of shape. During our visit, he said he planned to start taking more long walks. He also planned to do some volunteer work with local agencies. He had no plans to grow old early.

A person interested in health and long life might look at the numbers and switch his job to that of postman or bus conductor. But this might not necessarily help. First, how long has it been since you saw a postman on foot, or a double-decker bus? The era of physical passivity has engulfed us all. Second, another study published recently in the Metropolitan Life *Statistical Bulletin* noted that men listed in *Who's Who in America* lived longer than men in the general population. Seemingly, this disproved the active vs. sedentary theories. However, there was a hooker:

"The favorable mortality observed among the prominent men," read the report, "is believed to reflect in large measure their physical and emotional fitness for positions of responsibility." Thus, if you stay in good health you more likely will be in a position to make *Who's Who*.

The question becomes: How do you stay in good health? Do a hundred pushups each morning after arising? Bicycle to work? Run five miles during the lunch hour? Play an hour of tennis after you get home? Give up desserts and other foods that you like? Work out on a rowing machine before going to bed?

It gets down to the question of motivation. What motivates a man to change his pattern of living? One motivating factor could be a realization that unless he does, the odds are stacked against him. The prospects of a person's survival, in fact, may be reduced to numerical terms.

Take the dangers of heart disease, for example. The factors that appear to cause this ailment, particularly among the relatively young, have been readily identified by physicians such as Herman K. Hellerstein, M.D. Some years ago, Dr. Hellerstein and I collaborated on an article about coronary-prone characteristics. ("How Not to Have a Heart Attack," by Herman K. Hellerstein, M.D., with Hal Higdon; *The Kiwanis Magazine*, October, 1966). The doctor, one of the pioneers in the area of using exercise for preventive medicine, had identified 10 characteristics that increased your chances of dying from a heart attack. He theorized that an individual was more likely to develop premature heart disease if several of the following factors applied:

1. Male sex. Before the age of 40, men are 20-30 times more likely than women to suffer a heart attack. From age 40-49, the figure changes. Men are now only five times more likely than women to develop heart attacks, and three times more likely to die from the attack.

Something having to do with a woman's ovarian function apparently offers important protection from heart disease. After age 45, with the arrival of the menopause, women become increasingly prone to coronary attack—but still not to the same degree as men. Even at age 50-59, women run only one-third the risk of developing a heart attack and one-fifth the likelihood of dying from the attack.

Moreover, the more obviously masculine a person, the more coronary prone he is. Strange as it may seem (and for reasons not yet entirely understood by medical science), the more hair on a man's chest, the less hair on his head and the more masculine his body build, the greater are the odds against him.

2. Family history/heredity. If your father died early in life of a heart attack or if your brother also has had an attack, the odds are stacked against you, too. It is even worse if both parents have had an attack. In addition, if your family history includes diabetes, gout or high blood pressure, you may be even more susceptible. According to Dr. Hellerstein's studies at the Cleveland Work

Classification Clinic, 65% of young coronary victims have a family history of such diseases.

3. Cholesterol and diet. "Cholesterol" has become a dirty word to some members of the dairy and meat-packing industries. Cholesterol is a crystalline, fatty alcohol found in all animal fats, egg yolks, meat and shellfish. The human body also forms cholesterol.

Though some cholesterol seems to be necessary for health, too much can be dangerous. In relatively few people, blood cholesterol runs high because of metabolic diseases such as diabetes or thyroid conditions. More often, we find high concentrations of cholesterol in people who consume large amounts of animal fats, yet are not active enough to metabolize them. Compare this to burning ethyl gasoline in your automobile engine when regular or even kerosene would do. Eventually, the carbon deposits pile up inside the cylinders, and engine efficiency decreases.

Medical scientists have not yet determined exactly how high cholesterol content in the blood forms the plaques on the walls of the coronary arteries, though they do agree that these cholesterol plaques restrict the flow of the blood and lead to heart attacks. A man with a blood cholesterol level of over 300 milligrams per 100 cubic centimeters of serum is three times more likely to have his vital fuel lines clogged than if his cholesterol level were 200. The lower figure favors long mileage.

Studies show that in most people the level of cholesterol and other fats in the blood can be reduced and kept low by sticking to a low-calorie diet which substitutes polyunsaturated fats (mainly vegetable oils) for most animal fats.

4. Overweight. You might consider this a sub-category of diet since the eating of fatty foods that produces high cholesterol levels in the blood stream usually produces corpulence in the body and accompanying problems. The more extra weight you carry around, the greater the load on your heart and circulatory system. Obesity also means a larger likelihood of high blood pressure, high blood cholesterol, strokes and diabetes.

There is a sharp rise in the death rate (to 22%) for those even 10% overweight. If you are 20 or 25% overweight, the death rate for your category increases to 44 or 74%, respectively. An insurance study made by the Society of Actuaries in 1959 showed that 30 pounds of overweight shortens one's life expectancy by four years. On the optimistic side, obese people who bring their weight back to normal *and keep it there* have a normal death rate.

5. High blood pressure. In general, the higher the blood pressure, the greater the risk of having a heart attack or stroke. For example, if your systolic blood pressure were 160 or more, the risk of heart trouble would be four times greater than if it were 120 or less. Fortunately, this risk can be reduced. The mortality rate from high blood pressure between 1950 and 1960 showed significant decline of 50%, mainly because of new drugs that lower blood pressure. However, studies show that only 40% of those with high blood pressure are aware of it. And only 30% are under medical treatment.

6. Smoking. The dangers of smoking have generally been recognized, if not heeded, by most people. However, they usually associate these dangers with lung cancer. Yet smoking more than one pack of cigarettes a day will more likely cause their death through heart attack than through cancer.

The well-publicized Surgeon General's report announced that cigarette smoking was "causally related to lung cancer, and that male cigarette smokers had higher coronary artery disease rates than non-smokers, and that high mortality of cigarette smokers is associated with other disease of the heart and blood vessels." The report emphasized that "the harmful effects of smoking are indisputable and that deferment of remedial action cannot be justified."

In the population studies made in Chicago, Albany, New York and Framingham, Mass., cigarette smokers were found to be two times more likely to have a heart attack than non-smokers. However, the same studies have shown that by stopping the use of cigarettes, former smokers can reduce coronary risk. Pipe and cigar smokers can take comfort in the fact that they run no increased risk of heart attacks.

7. Reduced vital capacity. This relates to the maximum amount of air that a person can inhale and then exhale. If you have a low vital capacity, your risk of having a heart attack is about twice that of a person with a normal vital capacity.

Nobody knows exactly why. Cigarette smoking harms the sensitive lining of the air passages and reduces vital capacity. This is why track athletes, particularly long-distance runners, are warned by their coaches against smoking. Fortunately, vital capacity improves when cigarettes are discontinued.

8. Non-specific changes in the electrocardiogram. Whereas physicians once ignored this, several recent studies have shown that such changes (or indications of slight enlargement of the heart) increase the risk of heart attack 2 1/2 times over that of a person with a normal electrocardiogram.

9. Stocky, mesomorphic build. The person with a muscular or naturally athletic body structure is more susceptible to heart attack than the traditional endomorph (a chubby, soft person) or ectomorph (a thin, lanky person). Moreover, studies by Drs. Gertler and White indicate that a shorter person, particularly one below 5'8", is more likely to develop a heart attack than a taller one.

10. Lack of physical fitness. Regular physical activity, whether as a result of a person's occupation or his participation in sports or exercises, offers protection from heart attack. Men in occupations that keep them constantly on the move have a lower heart attack rate than sedentary people. In Dr. Daniel Brunner's study of Kibbutzim, Israel's collective agricultural settlements, sedentary workers had a rate of coronary disease three times higher than hard-working laborers, even though most other aspects of their lives were the same.

Though continuing studies indicated that maybe other factors contributed to the risk of an early heart attack—high blood level of uric acid (a chemical causing gout), stomach ulcers, chronic emotional stress and tension personality—Dr. Herman Hellerstein believed the 10 factors or danger signals above had definitely been linked to heart attack.

Various lists of coronary-prone characteristics are proposed, from time to time, by others. They vary in number from five to 15, but basically identify the same problems: heredity, diet, smoking, age and fitness. Thus, it becomes relatively easy to determine a person's proneness to heart attack. You might compare it to the way the Las Vegas gambler quotes odds.

Let us start with your age. If you are between 30 and 39, the odds against your developing a heart attack within the next 10 years are 30-1. If you are between 40 and 49, the odds are 14-1. If you are in your 50s, the odds are 8-1 that you will have a heart attack within the next 10 years.

If none or perhaps one of the 10 factors applies to you, the odds favor your not suffering a heart attack before age 60. If, for instance, the only factor that applies to you is that you are a male, and the other nine factors are absent, or weight, cholesterol and blood pressure are of low-normal value, the odds might be 140-1 or even 500-1 in your favor. But add high cholesterol, strong family history of heart disease and high blood pressure, and the odds would plummet to 100-1 or 50-1.

Then, if you smoked two packs of cigarettes a day, had a reduced vital capacity, were 15-30% overweight and, predictably, were physically unfit, the odds would be against you. They might go as low as 10-1, or even 3-1, or finally 3-4, until your chances of reaching age 65 would be slim indeed. Population studies have shown conclusively that combinations of two or more risk factors multiply a person's chances of developing coronary disease.

For example, if a middle-aged man has high cholesterol and high blood pressure, and if he smokes more than 20 cigarettes a day, his coronary proneness is more than 10 times greater than if he did not have these risk factors. If the same man has high blood pressure, high cholesterol and electrocardiographic abnormalities, his risk is seven times greater. If he smokes more than 20 cigarettes dialy, this risk is doubled!

Or look at it another way: If you statistically take a group of 1000 middle-aged men, eight will develop a heart attack each year. But if they each have three or more risk factors, as many as 40-50 of them will have a heart attack *each year*! And no doubt some of you who are reading this book can count eight, nine and even 10 factors in your case history.

Of course, we appear mechanistic when we examine a man with respect to a list of conditions and quote a set of odds on his ability to survive. But any insurance company does essentially that when it writes a policy requiring a man to pay an increased premium for being 10-15% overweight. The insurance people know the odds because they notice who dies early. It costs them money; that's why they notice.

Fortunately, you can improve the odds and expand your chances of survival by eliminating those elements in your physical makeup that lead toward heart attack. Two or three items probably cannot be done away with. If you're male, that's that. We could give you female hormones to slow down the rate at which your arteries age. But it's likely that you, like patients who have taken this medicine, would not relish the side-effects, such as enlargement of the breasts and reduced sexual performance. If you were born with a stocky, mesomorphic build you can't change it. Your family history of heart attacks, too, is irreversible. But you can change the family history of your son if you modify *your* way of living.

Consider some of the factors that can be eliminated. You can stop smoking. You can modify your diet by decreasing fat intake, so as to lower both cholesterol and weight. You can exercise to become physically fit. You can raise your odds of survival by simple acts of will-power.

For many years, Dr. Hellerstein directed a US Public Health Service-sponsored study program at the Jewish Community Center in Cleveland. Together with several associates at Western Reserve University, he conducted more than 500 coronary-prone men and 150 patients who have already been stricken with heart disease through a preventive program aimed at modifying the odds against them. The results were extremely encouraging. The mortality rate of the participants in the program was less than half of what might have been expected from their medical histories.

Basically, Dr. Hellerstein's program was simple. The men, mostly local businessmen, set aside one hour three or four times a week to participate in a program of physical exercise. They followed a low-fat diet to reduce their weight to within 5% of normal and to lessen cholesterol levels in their blood. The combination of dieting and exercise is a more effective way to reduce weight and cholesterol blood levels than either regimen alone. In addition, well-supervised exercise can lower blood pressure, increase vital capacity and improve the heart's response in exercise fitness tests, and often the electrocardiogram. And, of course, the total effect is improved physical fitness.

While working with Dr. Hellerstein in the mid-1960s on our article about coronary-prone characteristics, I visited the Jewish Community Center one noon and saw a "class" of 40 or 50 men working out. Their exercise program involved a half-hour of calisthenics, 15 minutes of running and walking, and a final 15 minutes of volleyball. Sometimes, they played handball or took part in any other physical activity that interested them. Some continued to jog; others substituted swimming for running. Not all participants in the program were allowed to exercise as vigorously as others. Instead of doing a dozen sit-ups, some might do six. All were under close medical supervision. In fact, several doctors participated in the program.

Dr. Hellerstein introduced me to a man named Sid who had visited his office one day several years before. Sid, 40 years old, weighed 320 pounds, which Dr. Hallerstein felt was at least 100 pounds too much. Sid was short of breath. He smoked continually. He could not walk to the corner without getting tired. He was the classic example of all that is wrong physically with middle-aged men.

Dr. Hellerstein gave Sid a physical examination, checked his family and medical history, and said to him, "The odds are 3-2 that you'll have a heart attack in the next five years.

Sid blanched, became irritated and asked Dr. Hellerstein how he had the nerve to make such a flat statement. Undoubtedly, Sid resented the fact that his doctor quoted odds on him the same way as a bookie quotes odds on a horse—and perhaps he should have. But Dr. Hellerstein simply was utilizing the knowledge gleaned during a lifelong quest for coronary-prone characteristics.

Two years later, through dieting and taking part in the program at the Jewish Community Center, Sid had cut his weight down to 210 pounds. Because of his increased physical activity, he found himself able to eat foods he had to ignore previously. Because of his improved health, he paid lower premiums on his life insurance—a recognition by at least one statistical source that his chances of staying healthy to a relatively old age had been significantly improved. He altered the odds in his favor. Not only did Sid show improvement in his physical fitness as tested scientifically, not only did he feel better, but he also insisted he was able to think better.

Later, Dr. Hellerstein offered a word of caution: "You can't just rush out for a quick run around the block. You might have some organic heart defect and by overloading your heart really upset the odds. Any return to physical fitness should be done in gradual steps and preferably under medical supervision. The important point is that if you really want to, you can re-stack the odds in your favor."

Unfortunately, while medical authorities like Dr. Hellerstein understood how to prevent heart attacks, doing lagged behind understanding. Many YMCAs and other clubs offer physical fitness programs, but in some areas facilities are few and far between. More often, it is the desire that is in short supply.

As for Sid, he still is alive and healthy a decade after I first met him. He had beaten the odds.

Recently, while researching this book, I returned to Cleveland to renew my acquaintance, after nearly a decade, with Herman K. Hellerstein, M.D. I wanted to know if the 10 coronary-prone characteristics he had identified for me earlier still served as a means of predicting heart disease. He said there were no major changes, only a few new wrinkles. For example, researchers know more about the effect of cholesterol today than before, but not as much as they still need to know. Some of the statistics have altered slightly, he said, but "if anything, the case is stronger today than before."

I visited him in his office on the fourth floor of Lakewood Hospital on the campus of Western Reserve University. When I arrived early one morning, I stopped first in the physiological laboratory nearby to watch several older men clad in shorts preparing themselves for an exercise test. Research continues.

During the testing, Dr. Hellerstein stopped by to say hello. He is a tall man with hawk-like features and curly, raven-black hair touched with grey at the temples. He wore half-glasses and a long, white physician's coat over grey trousers. Later, we moved into his book-filled office to talk. Among the books on the shelves was also written a book with John Naughton entitled *Exercise Testing and Exercise Training in Coronary Disease.*

A sign behind his desk announced, "I advise my patients not to smoke cigarettes."

Dr. Hellerstein peered at me over his half-glasses and talked about current research on heart disease. He cited several recent studies, some I had heard of, some of which I had not.

"What is very exciting," he said, "is there are now studies on newborn children made right after the baby has emerged from the womb and still is utilizing placental blood. Certain babies already have disturbances. They are people stigmatized by the dietary habits of their mothers during pregnancy. These are children who should require very stringent dietary control.

"We are victims of our heritages when it comes to health. There is the social heritage, which has to do with how you eat, how you sleep. Second, there is the chromosomal, or genetic, heritage: the chemical units you are endowed with at birth. The interplay between environmental and genetic affect our chances of survival.

"If you study children for coronary-prone characteristics, you often find children with elevated blood fats. Invariably, you find the parents have them, too. The quest for coronary-prone characteristics, which was focused 10 years ago on the middle-aged adults, now is being pushed back earlier. The problems that eventually surface at age 35, 40 or 50 have been there before, but have gone unrecognized."

Dr. Hellerstein has been doing a study on 750 medical students, drawing coronary profiles on them at age 21 or 22. He has found they already have a fair number of coronary-prone characteristics. For example, 68-70% had a positive family history of heart disease, diabetes, gout, stroke or premature atherosclerosis. Twenty-five to 30 per cent of them had cholesterol levels at least two standard deviations above normal. Fifteen per cent had high uric acid.

His study continued for fifteen years, however, and during this period the profile of medical students has changed. "We found in the past 15 years that the body weight of students has decreased," he said. "Medical students today are within 2-3% of the ideal weight. Smoking has dropped among potential doctors from 42% to 3%, so behavioral changes are taking place."

Dr. Hellerstein also commented on a subject I had discussed earlier with Dr. Kenneth Cooper: the drop in the mortality rate from coronary disease, beginning in 1968. He cited several reasons, one being improved methods of heart surgery, another being improved emergency techniques. Coronary care units have proliferated in hospitals, providing better survival odds.

But Dr. Hellerstein added, "While heart surgery does prolong life in people with certain kinds of lesions, the number of people operated on is small compared to the overall figure. The biggest percentage of people—55-60%—still die before they ever get to a hospital. So there must be other reasons if we are killing fewer of them.

"So the question is: Why has the mortality rate dropped? And it has dropped; the drop is real. Moreover, those people dying of heart attacks are dying at later ages than they once did.

"Each of us can take some credit. Blood pressure control has improved. There is no question that suppliers of food have found that there is money in low-fat, low-cholesterol diets. At one time, manufacturers could not mention low cholesterol in their ads; now they can. The number of cigarettes sold has increased, but not at the rate of the population increase.* Nicotine content of cigarettes has decreased, and that is having some effect. Willy-nilly behavior is changing. There is more public education, more information, more awareness of heart disease and the mechanism of death. And we don't want to forget the greater emphasis today on physical activities in all areas. There are now more bicycles than automobiles sold in the United States."

Dr. Hellerstein serves as president of the American Heart Association's affiliate in northwestern Ohio. It now has a program to train 520,000 people, or one out of every five persons in that part of the state, in basic cardiac-pulmonary resuscitation.

"That means that one person either in your household or next door will have training and can help you in an emergency," he said.

---

* Recent studies show that the number of cigarette smokers has increased to 58 million. But the percentage, when compared to the total population, has declined by 8%. Proportionately, fewer people are smoking today than yesterday.

"We know that even though the mortality rate has dropped, the disease has not been conquered," Dr. Hellerstein noted. "It still is the leading cause of death in America. There still are deficiencies in our thinking. President Ford's cancer budget was $800 million, his budget for heart disease only $300 million. Yet we know that in terms of the statistical impact, two or three times as many people die from heart disease as from cancer."

Dr. Hellerstein's concern is partly personal; he recently suffered a heart attack himself.

During one study of several thousand attorneys by Dr. Hellerstein and Ernest Friedman, M.D., they discovered that trial lawyers had no more heart disease than lawyers who did not practice in court. Seemingly, if you accept the principle that more stress is involved in a court room, this would contradict theories that stress causes heart attacks.

"Stress does not cause heart attacks," claimed Dr. Hellerstein. "Strain causes heart attacks. There has been a lot written about stress and the so-called Type A personality. But if a person is unable to cope, smokes too much, eats too much and has low self-esteem, he often develops heart disease. It may have a lot to do with social class."

Drs. Hellerstein and Friedman discovered that social class did have an effect in their study of attorneys. Lawyers who went to night law school had a higher heart attack rate than lawyers who went to Harvard, Yale, Princeton and the so-called other upper-class schools.

"The lawyers from those schools," Dr. Hellerstein explained, "were thinner, took more vacations, were more prudent with their life styles, had better health practices, were more physically active and had less heart disease."

But why? Dr. Hellerstein felt it went back to the importance of childhood influences. He explained, "The people who went to night law school undoubtedly were eating differently: hamburgers, french fries, all that junk-type food. By the time they got to be age 45 or 50, they were more overweight than other lawyers the same age accustomed to better health practices, despite the fact that they earned the same amount of money now and lived in the same communities."

Dr. Hellerstein has noticed differences in other professions, particularly his own. He stated, "Few cardiologists smoke, whereas general practitioners more often do. If you give a medical lecture to a group of general practitioners, they look different than a similar group of cardiologists."

He also noted that while lawyers who went to night law school have more heart disease, their sons (with better standards of living) do not. "They have the same genes," he said, "but they have less weight. They have more culture. There seems to be a gradual process of acculturation: the acquisition of certain patterns of behavior and style."

However, he did notice a decline in the health habits of one group: women. One coronary-prone characteristic is being male, but women are quickly approaching men in their ability to have heart attacks. In another few decades, the differences between the two sexes in this respect may disappear. Dr. Hellerstein put the blame on women's liberation:

"Women in being liberated, getting equal job opportunities, trying to get equal salaries, are doing equally stupid things that men did in the past, one of which is smoking cigarettes. The rate of cigarette smoking has declined among men but increased among women.

"They also take estrogen for birth control, becoming less womenly so they are infertile. Several studies in England and elsewhere show that women taking oral contraceptives have more intravascular problems, more clots in their veins, more clots going to their lungs, more strokes, more hemorrhages in the brain, more angina, more infarcts. In addition to that, in a certain number of people oral contraceptives set off high blood pressure by interfering with the angiotension. Even though the pills are withdrawn, hypertension continues. In essence, eating oral contraceptives is like eating a high-cholesterol diet. There is a rising specter of increasing occurrence of cardiovascular problems in women, who previously were 'protected' from coronary disease until they reached their menopause."

Dr. Hellerstein slowly shook his head: "So you can see that while we are making progress in certain areas, we are going backwards in others."

4

On the Edge of His Chair

One day in 1965, Gerald Smith, a Chicago-area commodities trader and insurance broker, arrived at his office in Lincolnwood, a suburb of Chicago at 7 o'clock in the morning. Smith, a wiry individual, once played basketball in high school despite being only 5'6" inches tall. Thirty-one years old, he continued to maintain his interest in physical activity, playing handball four or five times a week. As a handball player, he was intensely competitive—as he was in business.

Smith often worried about business and, as a result, slept fitfully. This morning he had awakened at 5:30, a half-hour earlier than usual. He rose, rather than lie in bed attempting further sleep, snatched a quick breakfast and left for the office.

Once there, he began experiencing signs of discomfort, belching frequently. He suspected he had a severe case of indigestion so decided to go downstairs to a restaurant and get some milk to coat his stomach. But the discomfort grew. Smith climbed into the back seat of his car, rolled down the windows and elevated his feet, but nothing helped. He felt chilled. He started sweating. Things began getting blurry. He looked up and saw a friend staring in the open car window at him. Smith had difficulty focusing on the friend, and wondered if it was part of a dream.

His friend appeared only by chance. He had parked nearby, glanced in Smith's car window and saw him suffering.

"My God, Jerry, what's the matter?" asked the friend. Smith could not reply.

The friend rushed him to the emergency room of Weiss Memorial Hospital. Gerald Smith was having a heart attack, although he felt no pain. "There was nothing like the binding wire across the chest you hear about," Smith recalls. "It was just a combination of nausea and sweating."

He remembers that, but little afterwards. Once in the hospital, he lost track of what was happening to him. His memory of the next 10 days is vague. His wife later told him he kept asking for hypodermic needles.

"I can remember getting them and noticing the door get blurry," Smith says. "I started to like that feeling."

He disliked what he learned later. He was stunned when the doctors told him he had experienced a heart attack. "I always considered myself in excellent condition," Smith insists. In addition to playing basketball in high school, he also ran the 660 on the track team. During the summer, for six years, he worked as a lifeguard for the Chicago Park District. He married, but did not (as too many people do) allow either his marriage or his business to interfere with his physical activities. He played handball to stay in shape. He disliked the thought of aging, of getting out of shape. He did not want to allow his body to deteriorate as had so many of his friends.

But there was that nervous, intense side to his personality. "In college they always used to call me, 'Smitty, the worrier,'" he admits. "If I had something to do tomorrow, I would spend the whole previous day and night worrying whether or not it might rain, and there was nothing I could do about it. I had what is known as a cardiac profile. A person with a cardiac profile is someone who, if somebody he plans to meet is a minute late, he's aggravated by it. He's always on time, never deviates from his schedule. He is, if anything, over-organized. Well, that was me."

This relates to the difference between Type A and Type B personalities, as classified by Drs. Meyer Friedman and Ray Rosenman. Type A individuals have driving, impatient personalities. They are extremely aware of the uses of time and continuously feel themselves under the pressure of meeting deadlines. They have greater heart attack risks.

Type B individuals, on the other hand, are more placid and have a lessened risk. Dr. Friedman first became aware of the time-consciousness of coronary patients when an upholsterer, hired to repair his office furniture, remarked that the chairs were worn mostly on the edges. The people waiting in Dr. Friedman's outer office literally had been sitting on the edges of their chairs!

Gerald Smith also had other coronary-prone characteristics. In a coronary risk estimate chart designed by Penn State University for the Central Pennsylvania chapter of the American Heart Association, one of the factors was sex. The scale for that category, in points, went from female (1), to female over 45 (2), to male (4), to bald male (5), to bald, short male (6), to bald, short, stocky male (7). The more points scored, the higher the individual's likeliness of developing heart disease. Gerald Smith can be recognized as a "bald, short, stocky male."

Yet he did not fit the pattern when it came to lack of exercise, which on the Penn State chart went, in points, from intense occupational and recreational exertion (1) to complete lack of exercise. Smith definitely was on the low point range of that scale—at least until he had his heart attack.

Under doctor's orders, he no longer could play handball. Being intensely competitive, he missed this opportunity to express himself athletically. He worried about being able to walk fast, let alone play a sport. He needed to report for blood tests once every 2 1/2 weeks to check against clotting.

"I thought I was going to be one of those rocking chair victims," he said. "I couldn't be the father I wanted to be—or the husband. I couldn't shovel snow. Things like having my wife carry the groceries from the car all the time were bugging the heck out of me. I became a second-class husband, father and citizen, and it wasn't my makeup to be that way."

He began hoping every night when he went to sleep that he would not wake up the next morning. He eventually began going to a psychiatrist, visiting him 26 times in 11 months. Depression is a common problem for heart attack victims.

Gerald Smith pondered the reasons for his heart attack. He was not overweight, although he had a dangerously high cholesterol level: around 450. He never smoked cigarettes. He did have a family history which hinted at possible cardiovascular problems, since his mother died at age 46 of a cerebral hemorrhage. His father, a former swimmer, had a mild heart condition but lived to age 66 before dying of virul pneumonia. Yet one grandfather was still alive at age 94 and in good condition.

"The only thing that aggravates him is when the Cubs lose," says Smith.

After several years of inactivity, Smith finally received permission from his physician to join an exercise class at the Lawson YMCA directed by Dick Woit. Woit's program, which attracted professional athletes as well as middle-aged businessmen, consisted of an intensive 45 minutes of almost unlimited push-ups, wind sprints and sit-ups.

Smith began the program by exercising at an easy level but soon increased his activity to where he was matching the achievement levels of others around him. His competitive nature was emerging once more. But he disliked the exercise program because it was boring and because it lacked the competitive aspect of other sports. He decided to return to handball.

"Handball is a game which is fun," Smith explains.

In 1973, several years after resuming handball play, he had troubles again, this time in the middle of a handball match at the Riviera Club. He began getting a feeling similar to the first attack and finally had to lie down on the floor. Fortunately, a physician present took his blood pressure and rushed him to Skokie Valley Hospital where his problem was diagnosed as a coronary insufficiency. The first attack had been diagnosed as a myocardial infarction, but the second attack was merely a matter of not enough blood getting through to the heart. Released from the hospital, he resumed playing handball as well as tennis.

"This is when things started coming together as to what was wrong with me," Smith explains. "I noticed each morning after driving to work that while walking from the car I would get a funny feeling in the area around my chin. But it would go away. Then I started noticing the same feeling during warmups to play tennis. It, too, would go away. I noticed that when I stopped warming up for a few minutes, the feeling would go away faster. But it still kept coming back again.

"It was explained to me later that I was suffered from angina. Every time the blood supply to the heart became insufficient, because of the blockage in the arteries, it would cause this funny sensation. Slowly, the blood would start circulating through other vessels to get around the blockage, what is known as collateral circulation. When the blood finally gets through, the pain starts subsiding."

At a tennis party one evening, Smith happened to meet a cardiovascular surgeon, Marlin Silver, M.D.*, a member of the staff of Rush-Presbyterian-St. Luke's Hospital on Chicago's near west side. One of Dr. Silver's colleagues was the physician who operated on Mayor Richard J. Daley, removing a blockage of the artery in his neck to improve circulation of blood to the brain and lessen the chance of a stroke. Dr. Silver performed a similar operations, but also specialized in coronary bypasses, a method of improving circulation to the heart.

The physician suggested that Smith's problems might be alleviated by such a bypass and asked him to visit the hospital for a stress test on a treadmill. Smith was on the treadmill for only a few minutes when Dr. Silver ordered it stopped. Smith's heart condition was such that it was dangerous to proceed, just as it would have been dangerous to continue playing handball.

Dr. Silver knew that Gerald Smith's cardiovascular system was what he describes as "severely compromised." He did not know how much. He ordered an angiogram, a test in which a tube is inserted into an artery (in Smith's case in the groin) so that a dye can be injected into the bloodstream. The dye then can be photographed by means of x-rays to determine how much blood can be carried to the heart.

The angiogram indicated that, indeed, Gerald Smith's circulatory system was severely compromised. Two of the coronary arteries leading into his heart were 100% blocked; the third was 80% blocked.

* Not his real name.

As Dr. Silver later explained, "Jerry Smith had major impairment of all the arteries, and his heart muscle was damaged from his previous heart attack. When we did the stress test, we weren't sure we would be able to help him despite his relatively young age. We feared he would be relegated to an inactive life."

But the angiogram indicated that his arteries were repairable by use of a bypass. There are three main arteries, and each of these arteries have branches. Atherosclerosis typically occurs in localized areas, usually where arteries branch, rather than equally throughout the cardiovascular system. Most of the narrowing occurs near the origin of the arteries, close to the heart. So although the arteries leading into Jerry Smith's heart were nearly totally blocked, the branches from them, in various other parts of his body, were relatively free of fatty deposits. If some means could be found for bridging the last few inches of blood flow into the heart, Smith might be able to return to normal activity.

Until the last few decades, patients as severely compromised as Gerald Smith were sent home with instructions to remain relatively inactive and wait for the inevitable closing of the final passage, with its accompanying massive heart attack followed by death. But in the mid-1960s, physicians developed a means of bypassing blocked arteries. Several physicians pioneered the technique, but the one who did the initial coronary bypass was a Dr. Favalero, then practicing in Cleveland, now returned to Buenas Aires. Among the people who have had bypasses are actor Walter Matthau and Michigan football coach Bo Schembechler.

While Marlin Silver, M.D., was in surgical training in 1970, he began learning how to perform bypass operations. There are perhaps 50,000 such operations performed in the United States each year, mostly at major medical centers.

Despite the operation's becoming routine because of its frequency, the coronary bypass remains a technically difficult procedure. Arteries are between one and two millimeters in size (approximately one-fortieth to one-twentieth of an inch). In order to join arteries, a surgeon must make 10-20 stitches.

"Each stitch is tiny and exact," says Dr. Silver. "One stitch can ruin an entire bypass."

In order to bypass the blocked coronary artery, Dr. Silver removed a saphenous vein from the inside of Gerry's left thigh. As yet, no artificial arteries have been developed capable of being utilized in a bypass operation, and only a few veins within the human body can serve as substitute coronary arteries. The saphenous vein is one such vein. Although it helps drain blood from the leg, there are additional deep veins that serve the same purpose. Once the saphenous vein is removed, those other veins assume its function, part of a backup system within the human body. The saphenous vein also serves well as a substitute coronary artery because of its elasticity, which makes it more capable of withstanding the pressures present in the arterial system.

Any operation, no matter how routine, contains risks. One risk in Gerald Smith's case was that his previously damaged heart might fail. It would be sustained during the lengthy operation by a heart-lung machine and other devices. But Dr. Silver worried that once the heart-lung machine was turned off following the operation, Smith's heart might not resume its normal function.

Dr. Silver estimated that Gerald Smith had an operative risk of 10-12%. The odds in his favor were about 9-1 that he would survive the operation. This compared to an operative risk on the average coronary bypass of about 5%. For a patient with no previous evidence of heart trouble, who was receiving a bypass for preventive reasons, the risk might be as low as 1%. For some patients with severely damaged hearts, the risk might be as great as 25-50%. With such odds, a surgeon probably would proceed with a bypass only if it was the last chance of saving that patient's life.

When coronary bypass operations were first performed, surgeons operated mostly on patients in their 50s and 60s. They did not operate on older patients, because the new technique seemed risky. They did not operate on younger patients for the same reason. Today, coronary bypass operations are being recommended for both older and younger heart patients.

"The state of the art has progressed," says Dr. Silver, "so with relative safety and confidence we may even recommend surgery to people who have not even had a heart attack yet." More patients in their 70s also are being given coronary bypass operations.

Dr. Silver admits to "dropoffs," patients who die within a year or two after surgery, but adds, "The dropoff in the post-operative patient is about a third of what it would be if those same patients did not have their surgery."

The operation on Gerald Smith proved successful. Ten days afterwards, he left the hospital. Forty-five days later, he began swimming, trying to get his chest muscles back in shape again. Four months following the operation, he began playing racquetball.

Gerald Smith believes he would have experienced much less trouble if he knew 10 years ago what he knows today. He advises, "Anyone over 40 who endeavors to go into any athletic activity, running or whatever, should go through a physical examination every year to check his blood pressure, check his heartbeat. He should also take a stress test, because that's a good indicator if you need an angiogram, which is a good indicator of whether or not you have some blocked coronary arteries, which seem to be more prevalent in people over 40. If I was a wealthy man, I would get on a soapbox all over the country and just talk about it.

"There are doctors completely against stress testing. They think it's dangerous. There are doctors completely against the angiogram for the same reason. There are doctors against the coronary bypass. But all I know is that I'm not experiencing that angina anymore. There supposedly is no definite data that a coronary bypass prolongs life. There is no way to prove that I'm going to live longer than if I had not been operated on, but I feel safe. I feel as though my blood is going all the way through my circulatory system and into my heart.

"There is a fellow who works for me in the next office who is 47, three years my senior. He had a coronary shortly after I did. He has a completely opposite life pattern. He does nothing athletically. He is extremely heavy. He drinks. Who's to say who is going to live longer?

"Right now, I am living a better life than I ever did before. I have complete confidence in my physical being. If something is going to happen, it's going to happen, but I don't think it would happen as much because of the surgery. What slows me down now is the fact that I'm 43, and I would start to slow down because of that anyway."

Presumably, the coronary bypass operation is the first step toward what might in coming centuries become a "Six-Million Dollar Man." Perhaps in some future medical era, artificial arteries can be devised as replacements for our actual coronary arteries, rather than using saphenous veins, which are in limited supply. Perhaps in some future era, such arteries can be replaced on schedule, like the oil filter on your automobile. Perhaps in some future era, we will have artificial hearts. We already have artificial pacemakers.

In the meantime, the Gerald Smiths of the world must learn to cope with their heart conditions, living life from one day to the next, hoping that the inevitable can be postponed. Jerry Smith comes off the racquetball court covered with sweat, a smile on his face, hoping that he can return to play racquetball one more time, then another time, then another time. He plays the game five days a week. He is very good at the game. He plays racquetball as though each game was his last, squeezing every drop of enjoyment he can out of life. Perhaps that is the way we should all play the game of life.

But there is no magic in the coronary bypass operation. Jerry knows it and is taking medication to lower his cholesterol level. He has reduced it from the 400s into the 300s. He is more careful with his diet now than before.

But Dr. Silver admits of him, "Jerry Smith is probably not your ideal patient." He follows orders grudgingly.

Several weeks after watching Jerry Smith demolish his partner in a game of racquetball, I spoke with Joan Ullyot, M.D., a San Francisco physician involved in sports medicine. Her husband Dan is a cardiovascular surgeon and performs coronary bypass operations. He also has done a study on patient mortality which seems to support the theory that, indeed, coronary bypasses do extend life rather than merely improve it.

"A coronary bypass operation doesn't cure you," Joan Ullyot told me. "It simply gives you another chance to do things better the second time around. The same disease is going to attack the substitute vessels unless you change your life style. It's an opportunity. You wrecked one set of arteries, so you have another set that are good for a couple more years. If you don't change, they, too, will clog up. It gives you a chance to stop smoking, start exercising, change your diet, change the stress level, whatever contributed to the clog-up the first time."

Joan described going to a party and meeting a young man on whom her husband had operated only a few months before. The young man, 28 years old, sat at the party smoking a cigarette.

Joan asked him, "Didn't they tell you at the hospital that smoking was bad for coronary patients?"

"Yeah," said the young man, "but I figure, easy come, easy go."

"Joan was appalled: "If you stop smoking, you'll have a better chance."

The young man attempted a smile: "I have a cholesterol level of 450, anyway. I might as well enjoy life while I can."

Joan Ullyot suspects that, coronary bypass or not, she may not see that individual at many future parties. "Obviously," she said, "his vessels are not going to last him very long. If he lives to age 30, he's lucky."

And I thought about Gerald Smith, a victim of his own Type A personality, still working, following his coronary bypass, in his two jobs a commodity trader and life insurance broker. When I first visited him in his office, I started to give my name to the receptionist, but Jerry was sitting nearby talking to one of his staff members, and he spotted me first.

"Two seconds," he said. "Two seconds." He help up two fingers to indicate how soon he would see me.

And he was sitting on the edge of his chair.

5

Targets

In the laboratory next to Herman K. Hellerstein's office at Lakewood Hospital in Cleveland, Barry Franklin, a physiologist on the doctor's staff, supervised an exercise on four middle-aged men. Each was clad only in shorts and running shoes. Three of the men had long, vertical scars almost from their necks to their navels, a sign of past bypass operations to correct clogged coronary arteries. For the last two years, they had taken part in exercise programs at the Cleveland and Lakewood YMCAs, and now they were visiting the laboratory for testing under a National Health Institute program to measure the extent of their recovery.

Barry Franklin helped an assistant tape leads to their chests. The leads connected to battery-powered telemetry devices attached to their waists. The devices sent electronic signals to a console at one end of the room displaying their heartbeats visually. At various positions around the room were a half-dozen exercise devices: (1) a small treadmill; (2) a rowing machine; (3) a step; (4) a large wheel turned by hand; (5) an exercise bicycle, and

(6) an exercise bicycle modified so it could be hand-cranked.

"Dr. Hellerstein believes that both the arms and the legs must be exercised to achieve fitness," Franklin explained. "One of his main concerns is that there is too much emphasis on cycling and jogging. The purpose of any fitness program should not be to pedal longer on your bicycle, but to enable a person to accomplish all his daily activities closer to maximum capacity."

With the telemetry units finally attached, the four men prepared for the test. They formed a small circle with Franklin in the center of the room. They opened with a brief warmup, but not the traditional routine of calisthenics. Franklin produced a medicine ball. He and the four others lay down on the carpet and raised their legs, passing the ball from one to the other. Then they got up and did another routine similar to drills basketball players perform, bending forward and rolling the ball around one leg, around the other, then passing it on.

Franklin previously studied under exercise physiologist Karl G. Stoedefalke at Penn State, who believes one way to make people exercise is to turn previously boring exercises into games. While at Penn State, Barry Franklin invented one game that involved kicking a soccer ball from telephone pole to telephone pole that transformed what previously had been a mile jog into a game of golf. Volleyball games under Stoedefalke's supervision were played allowing one bounce on the floor, making rallies longer for people with otherwise minimal athletic skills. Using such methods, Barry Franklin once led a class of 36 women with no dropouts and a 93% attendance rate over a three-month period.

But play with the medicine ball on this particular day was simply one means of getting his four test subjects warmed up for their series of exercises which were part of the NIH test. When Franklin said go, each of the four men stationed himself at one of the six devices and began to exercise. One walked on the treadmill. Another rowed the machine. The third wound the wheel. The last subject pedaled the exercise bicycle. None of the four seemed to be over-exerting himself; they carried on conversations while they exercised. At the end of four minutes, an alarm sounded and they received two minutes rest. Then each of the four rotated to a different station.

All during their exercise and rest period, they were being

monitored on the console, which not only displayed their electrocardiograph tracing but also the exact rate of their heart in beats per minute. Franklin called my attention to the stickers with each man's name on it pasted next to each of the heartbeat screens. The stickers predicted what he called "target" pulse rates for the four men of 111, 119, 105 and 116. The actual pulse rates were 105, 120, 105 and 117.

"That's not by chance," Franklin explained. "We know *exactly* what load to use to make them hit their targets."

Noting that the first man's pulse beat of 105 was slightly lower than his target of 111, he called to him to adjust the tension on the exercise cycle one notch higher for the last minute of exercise.

The term "target" was new to me, but as Barry Franklin explained, it referred to the exact level at which a person balances maximum benefit from exercise with minimum risk. Each man's target was not determined by chance, either, but only after a stress test to determine how fast his heart beat during maximum stress. Once that is determined, a target is set that can be between 70%-85% of maximum, but more often it is 75%.

The best way to determine your maximum heart beat is to take a stress test, but there is a way which an individual can predict his maximum pulse rate. The formula used is 220 beats minus your age in years. For example, my age is 45, which would mean my predicted rate (220 minus 45) would be 175. However, predicting your maximum rate can be imprecise, particularly with well-conditioned athletes. My actual rate, as measured on a treadmill, is 160.

To determine at which point you can safely train, you take 75% of that maximum pulse rate. In my case, that would be 120, the point at which I could expect to get optimum results from fitness training. If a person raises his heart rate much beyond that target level, it not only will provide him very little extra cardiovascular conditioning, but with some untrained individuals it could prove dangerous, even fatal. Yet to exercise below this target rate may not provide enough stress to improve an individual's fitness level.

Competitive athletes, of course, often train at levels near 95% of their maximum heart rate. They not only are interested in training their cardiovascular system to work efficiently (which can be done through long, slow distance running, what Joe Henderson labels

"LSD" training), but they also are training their muscles to work efficiently. Thus a four-minute miler may run frequent quarter-miles at race pace (60 seconds per lap) to learn the rhythm of his race. In doing so, he would exceed the so-called cardiovascular target level of 75%. But most heart patients do not run four-minute miles, so they exercise at a much lower level.

The interesting point about target training is that exercise physiologists now can prescribe levels of activity for cardiac patients interested in improving their fitness to prevent further heart attacks.

After the four individuals finished their test, I sat down with Barry Franklin in his office next to the exercise room. He described the test study involving 170 men in the Cleveland area: half in an exercise group, half in the control group. It was hoped the study would document changes in fitness and also document future events, including morbidity and mortality. The four men exercising in the lab that morning were members of the exercise group, having been chosen randomly for that group. If early results are any indication, that may prove to be a fortunate choice for them.

Of four deaths in the two years since the four-year program began, three were in the control group, only one in the exercise group. Barry Franklin concedes that, considering the small number, the results are not yet statistically significant. Similar studies are going on in four other centers.

"If we continue to experience mortality at that ratio, and if all the other centers report three-to-one and four-to-one figures, it may mean something," he said.

In the meantime, the capacity of the exercise subjects under his supervision to accomplish work—a value that some researchers refer to as maximum oxygen uptake—has increased by an average of 20%.

Barry Franklin, however, talks in terms of "mets," an abbreviation for "metabolic cost of activity." One met is the energy a person expends at rest.

Franklin explained, "The average person takes in 250 milliliters of oxygen a minute at rest. If you divide that by his average body weight in kilograms, it gives you 3.5 milligrams of oxygen per kilogram per minute. If we were to put you on a treadmill, walking at three miles per hour up a 17.5% grade, it would require 10 mets. Your ability to maintain that pace would depend on your capacity to work at that level."

A well-conditioned athlete might have a work capacity as high as 20 mets. A moderately fit individual might be closer to 10 mets. A heart patient's capacity could be as low as five mets.

A person's ability to raise his met level depends partly on his initial fitness. One woman in the program showed a 42% improvement. She exercised faithfully five days a week and lost 30 pounds doing so. Her met capacity went from eight to 11.5.

Barry Franklin raised his two palms before his face, one slightly higher than the other. "If your met capacity is here (indicating the top palm), and your daily tasks require this much reserve (indicating the slightly lower palm), you have very little reserve," he said.

He raised the upper palm. "But if your met capacity is up here, you have plenty of reserve capacity. People ask, what is fitness? It's having the reserve capacity to perform daily tasks."

In the early predawn hours of a wintry morning on the north side of Chicago, people jog. They are mostly men, but some are women. They run in circles around the basketball court in the gymnasium of North Park College. Signs on the wall exhort the Vikings (nickname for that college's athletes) to charge, to fight, to *win!* But these are not Vikings, either figuratively or imaginatively. These are heart patients in an exercise program run by Noel D. Nequin, M.D., director of the Cardiac Rehabilitation Center at nearby Swedish Covenant Hospital.

Some of the joggers move swiftly, effortlessly, in groups of two, three, four or more. By their easy conversation while running, it seems apparent that they feel no stress. Others move more slowly, gently, almost *gingerly*. Still others walk.

At regular intervals, different individuals disengage themselves from the steadily moving stream of joggers and stop in the gym's southeast corner to stare up at a clock on the wall. They clutch their throats and stare upwards for precisely 10 seconds. Then they rejoin the stream—or move to the locker room to shower and go home.

The throat clutching actually is pulse taking. The joggers feel the carotid artery or wrist, count the number of heartbeats in 10 seconds, and that gives them their pulse rate. It tells them if they are on target. Each of the heart patients jogging (or walking) in the gym has been given a prescription by Dr. Nequin, which includes a 10-second target pulse rate to achieve through exercise. The target pulse is 75% of their attained maximum pulse rate as determined by a stress test in his laboratory.

"We found that giving one single target pulse was better than giving two numbers," explains Dr. Nequin. "We used to give a lower limit of 70% and an upper limit of 85%. What happened was that most of the heart patients exercised to their upper limit rather than their lower one. So now we just make 75% the target."

Dr. Nequin is among the exercisers circling the gymnasium floor. He is a short man, 39 years old, with olive complexion, long, straight, black hair, glasses and an infectious smile that makes you immediately want to like him. As he jogs, he moves smoothly, gracefully, but not swiftly.

"I am not a competitive runner," he says.

We had arrived at the gymnasium a 7 a.m. and soon after that hour began an exercise routine of 5-10 minutes of stretching led by Donald R. Timm, an exercise physiologist and program coordinator for the Cardiac Rehabilitation Center. That warmup completed, we began to jog in a clockwise direction, talking as we went. About 15 or 20 minutes into the workout, a second group materialized to start another warmup before also beginning to jog. We continued clockwise until around 7:30 when someone shouted, "reverse," and we went counter-clockwise.

As time passed, people stopped jogging, one by one, until near 8 o'clock there was only Noel, myself and a handful of others circling the gym. This last group included Joe Friedman who several years before had a coronary bypass operation, began jogging as a form of preventive rehabilitation and now is beginning to branch out into participation in competitive distance runs.

More or less spontaneously, we stopped. As we did, Dr. Nequin announced that he perceived his pulse to be about 22 (for 10 seconds) and clutched his throat while staring at the clock. "Twenty-two," he announced triumphantly. Multiplied by six, that meant his heart was beating at a rate of 138 beats per minute, or right on target.

He asked mine. "Eleven," I announced, or 66 beats per minute.

Noel's eyebrows arched briefly. "That's because you're a competitive runner," he stated, and grabbed me by the throat, not from anger but from scientific curiosity. He nodded to indicate my count had been correct.

Though Noel D. Nequin, M.D., does not classify himself as a competitive runner, having run for 45 minutes, conversing continuously and showing no signs of distress or fatigue, he displayed a fitness level higher than perhaps 99% of the American public.

As for my fitness level, I simply run faster. Athletic efficiency or ability bears no direct relationship to general health. It is what you do with that ability that counts.

Noel Nequin was born in the town of Iloilo in the Philippines on Dec. 9, 1937. "I was a non-athlete, a bookworm," he explains. "In high school and college, I took roll call rather than get out on the athletic field. I assigned work for other people rather than do it myself."

He attended medical school at Far Eastern University in Manila, spending two years as a resident physician at Clark Air Force Base before coming to the United States in 1963. He trained in internal medicine and cardiology at Swedish Covenant Hospital and Hines Hospital in Chicago until 1969, when he established a private practice at the former place.

In working with heart patients, he soon began to feel the need for a standardized rehabilitation program involving exercise. He became aware of the work of others in this field, including Dr. Hellerstein in Cleveland, Dr. Cooper at the Aerobics Center in Dallas, Dr. John L. Boyer in San Diego, Dr. Robert Bruce in Seattle, Jack Wilmore, then at the University of California in Davis, Philip K. Wilson in La Cross, Wisc., Dr. L. Loring Brock in Denver and Dr. Terrence Kavanagh in Toronto.

Dr. Nequin explains, "Many physicians, either through formal studies or informal consultation with people in the same field, came to the consensus that heart patients recuperate faster with exercise than without it."

In Dr. Nequin's program, a patient recovering from a heart attack is given a prescription, which tells him what exercise to take rather than what medicine to take. "It's like any other form of medication," he explains, "where you identify type of medicine (such as aspirin) and strength (such as two grains) and frequency (such as every four hours)."

Dr. Nequin's exercise prescriptions, determined only after a stress test in the laboratory, include: (1) type; (2) intensity; (3) duration, and (4) frequency. For example, a heart patient might be told: (1) to cycle; (2) fast enough to raise his pulse to 140; (3) 30 minutes per session; (4) three times (minimum) a week. The prescription also suggests a warmup and cooldown period of 5-10 minutes each. The most important ingredient in the prescription is the target pulse, and presumably if Dr. Nequin and his associate, Don Timm, have prescribed properly, the patient will complete his exercise period on target. As the patient's fitness increases, the prescription will be adjusted to permit additional exercise. The target remains the same, but the amount of exercise required to reach target becomes greater. Said another way, the patient can exercise longer or more vigorously before being warned by elevated pulse levels to quit. Actually, patients write their own prescriptions in that they control dosages by monitoring their pulse rates during exercise, as the joggers in the gym did each time they paused by the clock.

"It takes practice," explains Dr. Nequin, "but eventually they are able to perceive their heart rates without taking their pulses. They can predict their pulses during exercise by knowing how they feel. It is a matter of experience. This is when we allow them to play tennis, swim, go hiking and engage in other active sports, because they know when to stop."

Another computation figured into the prescription is a person's met level, which relates to his maximum oxygen uptake. This, too, is determined during a stress test. A person with a maximum met capacity of 12 can safely perform an activity that requires nine mets. This would include heavy labor, if he were working. This also would include fencing, non-competitive handball and vigorous basketball, if he were exercising. If the individual's maximum met level were 10, however, his safe level would be close to seven, and he should not engage in those activities. At the other end of the fitness scale, a person with a maximum level of 12 would not be able to use golf as a sport for conditioning, because the level of activity for that sport (two or three mets) is too low to affect his fitness positively.

How often a person exercises also is an important part of the prescription. Exercise, like uranium, has a half-life. Physiologists have computed the half-life for exercise as 2 1/2 days.

"In order to maintain your fitness level," explains Dr. Nequin, "you must reinforce your body with exercise every 60 hours. When the prescription exercise idea became popular, we used to say a minimum of three days a week was necessary. Now we talk more about four days a week, because that comes closer to the ideal of never resting more than 60 hours (2-1/2 days) between exercise. In order to maintain your fitness level, you want gentle hills rather than tall peaks and deep valleys. Weekend athletes are nowhere near as fit as individuals who do maybe one-third or one-fourth as much, but on a more regular basis."

Prescribing exercise is extremely important in ministering to high-risk heart patients for whom guidelines on stressful activity must be extremely precise: that is, too much exercise may kill them, but too little exercise may also kill them!

Dr. Nequin believes that apparently healthy individuals also can benefit from target training: "If we tell them to do nine-minute miles, they might find that more pleasant and enjoyable than if they sought their own level, did 7:30 miles, and hated it. For the 'apparently' healthy individual, it might be crucial to identify the comfortable level at which they can exercise."

When Dr. Nequin uses the word "healthy," he usually precedes it with the adverbial modifier, "apparently." And to further set off that modifier, he raises two fingers of each hand and makes slashes in the air—slash, slash—to indicate quotation marks. He feels that what the general population (and many physicians, unfortunately) perceive as good health in this country is woefully inadequate. A person who others consider healthy may have a metabolic capacity so low that even walking up stairs may strain his heart. As a result, individuals categorized as, (1) apparently healthy, may pass quickly into the categories of (2) heart patients or (3) deceased.

Dr. Nequin spends most of his time working with people in that middle category. He has 150 participants in his morning exercise programs, some who come Mondays, Wednesdays and Fridays, some who come Tuesdays, Thursdays and Saturdays, and some who come a combination of days.

"That is nowhere near the size of some programs," he admits. "Honolulu has somewhere near 450. But it's a dent in Chicago. When we started in 1971, we were the first in this city. Now there must be three or four similar programs in the Chicago area, and I expect more to start in the next few years."

During the winter, Dr. Nequin's group uses the North Park College gymnasium, and when the weather warms, they move to that college's outdoor running track, midway between gym and hospital.

Presently, Swedish Covenant Hospital is considering a million dollar fund-raising campaign to construct a specific exercise facility, similar in some respects to Dr. Cooper's Aerobics Center in Dallas. North Park College also has expressed an interest in some shared facility, although Dr. Nequin worries whether non-competitive patients should mix with possibly competitive students—or whether non-competitive students should mix with possibly competitive patients. Nevertheless, he feels many preventive medicine exercise facilities will be constructed in the next few decades as people become more aware of their benefits.

"The program can only serve the people who really feel a need for it," concedes Dr. Nequin. "The people who feel this need are those who have been identified as having heart disease. The motivation is there. The need is there. Whereas other apparently normal individuals can get very presumptive if they feel they are normal. What some people consider 'normal'" — and again Dr. Nequin makes slashes in the air—"may not necessarily be healthy."

Perhaps the most unfortunate part about programs such as Dr. Nequin's and many of the others across the United States, is that they mostly serve people *after* they have heart attacks, or at least have symptoms of coronary artery disease.

Several weeks after my jog with Noel Nequin in the North Park gym, I visited him in his laboratory on the fourth floor of Swedish Covenant Hospital. The laboratory contained two treadmills, along with various other diagnostic devices for measuring response under stress.

Each morning, Dr. Nequin and Don Timm test 5-6 individuals. That morning, they tested a person who previously had severe chest pains but waited a week before seeing his doctor. The doctor hospitalizied him for seven days, but the man displayed no symptoms. Released, the man reported for a stress test to Dr. Nequin, who still saw no symptoms but uncovered what he described as "responses more severe than clinically identifiable."

Dr. Nequin noticed evidence of ischemia on the man's electrocardiograph tracing. Ischemia is a temporary lack of blood supply to an organ or tissue, in this instance to the heart. This is not necessarily considered cause for alarm, provided it goes away five or 10 minutes after termination of exercise. The man's ischemia, however, remained evident 35 minutes after the treadmill test. He seemed a likely candidate for a second heart attack, perhaps a fatal one. Dr. Nequin recommended an arteriogram to determine whether or not coronary arteries were blocked. The eventual treatment might be a coronary bypass followed by an exercise regimen to prevent further blockage.

The five or 10 minutes during which ischemia should disappear from an electrocardiograph relates to Dr. Kenneth Cooper's theory that five or 10 minutes after exercise a person's pulse rate should recover to below 100 beats. If not, the exercise may have been too severe.

Another more subjective way to determine exercise severity is the so-called talk test. If you can carry on a conversation while jogging, or performing another fitness activity, you probably are undergoing minimum stress. Some people use this talk test as a means of defining the difference between jogging and running: if you no longer can talk, you must be running. But this varies greatly, depending on the condition level of individuals. Many competitive runners, including myself, can carry on conversations while running near five-minute mile pace in long-distance races.

As Dr. Nequin explains, "The unfit individual will hit his target sooner than the fit individual, so he has to slow down sooner."

(Of course, the person carrying on a conversation while exercising may be doing too little to improve or maintain his fitness. Thus the need for a prescription, including a target.)

Thirteen laps around the North Park Gymnasium equals one mile. A person whose prescription tells him to go at 60 seconds per lap can probably do it walking. A person prescribed to do 50 seconds per lap will find himself jogging. Dr. Nequin says that when you cover laps in 35 seconds you are running.

But often when an individual reaches that level of fitness, he finds circling around a gymnasium floor increasingly less stimulating and moves to the outdoors, running long distances in the parks and on the roads regardless of the weather. He runs in snow, rain, cold, heat, sweat on his brow, a smile on his face. That person has become a victim of positive addiction. He also will have crossed the bridge from rehabilitative jogger to competitive runner, a bridge that Dr. Nequin does not necessarily feel needs to be crossed, although he might be considered poised at least at the toll gate himself.

"I started running about three years ago," he confesses, "more from the influence of what I saw in my patients, rather than being an inherent runner myself. Once I started running, people began to suggest I try running a marathon. I resisted the idea at first, but then succumbed to it. A lot of other physicians I know, particularly cardiologists, run marathons.

"They told me the best place to start was the Honolulu Marathon, because unlike the Boston Marathon, there is no qualifying time and the officials always wait for the last runner to come in. I began training for the Honolulu Marathon in February 1975, and that December finished the race in 4:10.

"Then to keep myself motivated, because I am basically noncompetitive, I trained last year for the Boston Marathon.* I perceived my training, and one month before Boston I wrote on a piece of paper what I thought I could do. I wrote down 3:50, and I actually finished in 3:51." Noel smiles. "It was a hot day."

A person lying in the coronary care unit of Swedish Covenent Hospital, however, cannot visualize the finish line of the Boston Marathon, the thousands of people lining each side of the street before Prudential Center, cheering each competitor as he or she crosses the line. That patient only worries whether he will survive from one minute to the next. Once out of bed—and heart patients today get out of bed much sooner than they did 20 years ago—he begins a steady rehabilitation program, often beginning with 25 tottering steps to the end of the hospital corridor, then 25 back.

If Dr. Nequin becomes involved in such a patient's rehabilita-

---

* Although most runners must run under three hours to qualify for the Boston Marathon, 3:30 for people over 40, the American Medical Joggers Association runs a special section at Boston for physicians with no standard, other than an M.D. degree.

tion, he evaluates the patient's capacity for exercise and identifies symptoms. During the first week out of bed, a heart patient is not allowed to elevate his pulse more than 15 beats per minute. After a week, he must keep his beat during minimal exercise within 25-30 beats of resting pulse. Easy walking is all that is allowed for the first eight weeks after a heart attack.

"It takes around six weeks for the heart muscle, if it is damaged, to firm into a good scar," explains Dr. Nequin. "With exercise tests, we can determine how soon it is safe to begin exercise."

One method is to have a cardiac patient carry a Holter recorder for a period of 24 hours. This records his pulse levels on a miniature tape. Recent research has indicated that certain activities provide much less stress than physicians formerly believed. For example, resumption of normal sexual relations is no longer considered as dangerous. Previous studies indicated that sexual relations resulted in pulse rates of 160-180. But research by Dr. Hellerstein and others showed that the peak pulse rate for most individuals was 117.

After eight weeks, the cardiac patient may enter an exercise program such as the one of Dr. Nequin. "The first few weeks usually consist of walking," he explains. "Jogging is added only after an exercise test and only if we identify that the pace on the prescription is jogging."

Alas, only a small percentage of the heart patients in Chicago become involved in exercise programs. There are two reasons, the first being motivation.

"They might be motivated into going through a testing and exercise program, but personal interest—or lack of it—and job demands prevent them from coming regularly," Nequin says.

Most people who do become involved in the Swedish Covenent program stay in it, often developing new friendships, new interests, supported by others around them. It is a bit like Alcoholics Anonymous, except they have given up heart attacks instead of alcohol. It becomes less oppressive rising an hour earlier to exercise in a gym if you know others in your peer group are doing the same. It is less a case of misery loves company than it is a case that company prevents misery. The dropout rate in Dr. Nequin's program is about 10% after two months.

But a more pernicious reason why cardiac patients do not get involved with exercise programs is that their physicians fail to refer them to such programs. Many physicians still do not believe in exercise as a means of preventive medicine. Dr. Nequin cautiously admits the accuracy of that statement:

"There is some reluctance on the part of the medical community concerning this recent change from bedrest treatment of heart attacks to early mobilization." He pauses as though awaiting a lightning bolt of colleagal displeasure to strike him. None striking, he continues, "For physicians who don't have too much personal background in exercise, and that once included myself, it may be difficult for them to understand the present stage of cardiac rehabilitation."

Or they refuse to change! Dr. Nequin recently lectured in a small town in downstate Illinois. Afterwards, an older cardiologist approached him.

"I don't object to your program," explained the cardiologist, "but I've been telling my patients: stay in bed six weeks and not return to work for three months. If I tell them they now can get out of the hospital in three weeks and go back to work in 6-8 weeks, that makes me look like a liar. I'd be losing face."

So instead of looking like a liar, that physician, and many others like him who resist change, go on lying to their patients. Dr. Nequin admits that most referrals to his program are from relatively young doctors in their 30s. Rarely does he get referrals from physicians in their 60s. This eventually will change. Doctors in their 30s soon become doctors in their 60s. And so American medicine boldy steps toward the future in fighting heart disease.

Dr. Nequin seems willing to wait, but he may not need to. "With more and better education for the public concerning heart disease and prevention," he says, "more patients are pushing their doctors to allow their involvement in programs such as these. My own personal testimony as a physician is that I knew very little about running or rehabilitation through running until I got acquainted with non-physician runners. There is a lot to learn from these runners, and I think I have grown professionally, not only from reading about running, and looking into running and other exercise activities, but more from learning what other people have experienced.

Energy Expenditures in Different Sports

	Occupational	Recreational
1½-2 mets*	Desk work Auto driving Typing	Standing Walking (strolling 1 mile per hour) Playing cards
2-3 mets	Auto repair Radio, TV repair Janitorial work Typing, manual Bartending	Level walking (2 miles per hour) Level bicycling (5 miles per hour) Billiards, bowling Golf (power cart) Canoeing (2½ miles per hour) Horseback riding (walk)
3-4 mets	Brick laying, plastering Wheelbarrow (100-lb. load) Machine assembly Trailer-truck in traffic Welding (moderate load) Cleaning windows	Walking (3 miles per hour) Cycling (6 miles per hour) Horseshoe pitching Volleyball (6-man noncompetitive) Golf (pulling bag cart) Archery Sailing (handling small boat) Horseback (sitting to trot) Badminton (social doubles)

*1 met = oxygen uptake of about 3.5 ml./kg./min. or approximately 1.1 kcal./min.; figures here include resting metabolic needs.

Reprinted from Fox, S.M., Naughton, J.P., and Gorman, P.A: Physical activity and cardiovascular health. III. The exercise prescription; frequency and type of activity. Mod Concepts Cardiovasc Dis 41:6, June 1972.

	Occupational	Recreational
4-5 mets	Painting, masonry Paperhanging Light carpentry	Walking (3½ miles per hour) Cycling (8 miles per hour) Table tennis Golf (carrying clubs) Dancing (foxtrot) Badminton (singles) Tennis (doubles) Many calisthenics
5-6 mets	Digging garden Shoveling light earth	Walking (4 m.p.h.) Cycling (10 m.p.h.) Canoeing (4 m.p.h.) Horseback (posting to trot) Ice or roller skating (9 m.p.h.)
6-7 mets	Shoveling 10 min. (10-lb. load)	Walking (5 m.p.h.) Cycling (11 m.p.h.) Badminton (competitive) Tennis (singles) Folk (square) dancing Light downhill skiing Ski touring (2½ m.p.h.; loose snow) Water skiing
7-8 mets	Digging ditches Carrying 80 lbs. Sawing hardwood	Jogging (5 m.p.h.) Cycling (12 m.p.h.) Horseback (gallop) Vigorous downhill skiing Basketball Mountain climbing Ice hockey Canoeing Touch football Paddleball

	Occupational	Recreational
8-9 mets	Shoveling 10 min. (14-lb. load)	Running (5½ m.p.h.) Cycling (13 m.p.h.) Ski touring (4 m.p.h.; loose snow) Squash racquets (social) Handball (social) Fencing Basketball (vigorous)

10-plus	Shoveling 10 min. (16-lb. load)	Running:
		  6 m.p.h. = 10 mets
		  7 m.p.h. = 11½ mets
		  8 m.p.h. = 13½ mets
		  9 m.p.h. = 15 mets
		  10 m.p.h. = 17 mets
		Ski touring (5-plus m.p.h.)
		Handball (competitive)
		Squash (competitive)

Part Two: ATHLETICS FOR OLDSTERS

6
"They're Not Runners; They're Too Old"

In 1972, I visited England along with several hundred other Americans, Canadians and Australians to compete in the International Veteran's Athletics Meeting, a track and field meet for athletes 40 and older. It was the first major international meet for Master runners and would be followed three years later by a *world* championships in Toronto.

We stayed in a hotel in downtown London. During the nearly one week spent in that city, I watched each day as workmen demolished a building across the street from our hotel. I was fascinated by the precision with which they worked. They pecked at the masonry with picks and sledges. Bit by bit, pieces of the old structure came unstuck to crash below.

I could not help comparing that building to the human body. The body takes time to construct, decays gradually. Eventually, along come the wreckers to dismantle it brick by brick.

One of the attractions, however, of veterans' athletics (what in the United States is called "Masters track") is that you can beat that schedule. By conditioning yourself—and even competing as in youth—you can become younger physically and spiritually while aging chronologically. It is almost as though, after the workmen had finished their day's demolition, a new crew of masons appeared at night to raise the building higher than the day before. But this only postpones the inevitable. Sooner or later, the building tumbles to the ground.

I thought of that as, day after day, I observed the workers pecking away at the building. Eventually, it would be gone. Yet as I watched from the window of my London hotel, I could not help thinking, again, that back in the United States a tractor crane would have swung its iron ball, and the building would have fallen in hours instead of weeks.

Our group of Master athletes, every one of us over 40, formed an interesting group. There was Roland Anspach, for example, who worked for General Motors in Dayton, Ohio. When he turned 40 he began to run even though he never had competed in track before.

"It was something I always had wanted to do," Roland explained to me one day. "At first, I trained while delivering my son's paper route so the neighbors wouldn't think me crazy."

After six months' preparation, Roland entered his first race, a Masters mile at Ohio University, and wheezed across the line in 5:50. Four years later, he ran on a 24-hour relay team, averaging 5:27 for 25 separate miles. He no longer delivered newspapers.

"The neighbors are used to me now," he said.

There was Thane Baker who competed in the Olympic Games in 1952 and 1956, winning silver medals in the 200 meters and a gold medal in the 400-meter relay. He retired following his second Olympic appearance but came out of retirement after turning 40 to run 100 yards in 9.8 seconds. A lot had changed during his retirement, including tracks, once all cinder, now mostly hard, all-weather combinations.

Flying across the Atlantic, Baker commented to me, "You know, I've never run on an all-weather track before. I don't even own a pair of shoes with short spikes yet!" When he landed in London, one of his first priorities was finding a sporting goods store to buy some.

Rudy Friberg of San Diego competed in the pole vault. Several decades earlier, he had vaulted for Fresno State, clearing 13'6" and earning All-American status. That was back in the bamboo pole era. He was competing now on a fiberglass pole and wondering if this might offer him the opportunity to better even his collegiate personal best. He fell several feet short of his goal, but Roger Ruth of Victoria, British Columbia, soared well above 15 feet, which had he accomplished it in his youth would have earned him an Olympic medal.

There was Jim O'Neil of Sacramento, Calif., who had attended the University of Miami in Florida where he became number three man on a cross-country team that ran only one race a year. He was racing faster at age 47 than he did in college.

"There always have been opportunities for older distance runners," O'Neil commented to me one afternoon, "but the good thing about the Masters program is it gives the sprinters and jumpers a chance to compete again."

One well-known individual the sport attracted was Alan Cranston, who ran on the track team at Stanford University in the late 1930s and three decades later became a US Senator from California. This lofty position failed to dampen his enthusiasm for sports competition, however. Most politicians seem content to sit in the stands and watch others perform. They throw out the first ball at major league baseball games and such. But Sen. Cranston appeared one winter to run the 50-yard dash at a San Francisco indoor track meet in a special race for men over 50. At the starting line, he removed his sweat pants—and his shorts along with them. The exposure did not seem to harm his next re-election campaign.

Cranston ran on one of our sprint relay teams in London. After the race he came up to me in the stands and asked, "How did I look?"

"You looked great!" I told him.

The senator persisted: "No, how did I look against the other runners on my leg?"

While I had watched Alan high-stepping down the back straightaway, I could not recall the other runners around him. But I had a bit of the politician in me as well. "You ate them up!" I announced.

A broad smile crossed the face of the senior senator from California.

Alphonse Juilland, head of Stanford's linguistics department, also traveled with us to Europe. As a boy, he competed in the sprints in his native France, but World War II halted a promising athletic career. He began jogging again at Stanford, got to know members of the track team and attended the West Coast Relays to watch Bill Toomey perform.

The program featured a 100-yard dash for senior runners, and several of Alphonse's students pulled him out of the stands, demanding he compete. Wearing a borrowed pair of shoes, he placed second, pulling a leg muscle while doing so. But the competitive bug had struck. Alphonse set his goal at running 11.0 for 100 yards, and while 50 years old he ran that distance in 10.5 seconds.

While traveling by boat from Helsinki to Stockholm, one evening I questioned Juilland about the dangers that older athletes faced by taking part in an explosive event like the 100-yard dash. Older men traditionally have raced in long-distance events. Clarence DeMar won the Boston Marathon seven times and continued running that event until age 65. But no sane man would attempt a marathon—or even a mile—without training. Because 100 yards is so short, there remained the danger that once-fast athletes might jump into such a race with inadequate preparation and injure, or even *kill*, themselves.

"I'll admit some danger," Alphonse replied. "But older sprinters must prepare for competition by becoming long-distance runners first—then working down to shorter distances at faster speeds. They probably should obtain a thorough medical checkup before starting—not just a regular electrocardiogram, but a *dynamic* electrocardiogram in which a trained physiologist monitors the heart under exercise."

"It's hard enough to find a doctor with time enough to take your temperature these days much less give you a thorough exam," I commented.

"True," Alphonse admitted. "But I think maybe we harbor too many fears about what men past 40 can accomplish. We age ourselves prematurely by thinking old. Take Adolfo Consolini. At age 47, he still held the Italian record in the discus and continued to throw. He was the best thrower in his country and one of the best in the world. But according to Italy's athletic rules, nobody past the age of 45 could compete. So Adolfo had to join a Swiss club and compete in his home country as a foreigner."

I understood what Alphonse meant. The average citizen does *not* expect people in their 40s, 50s, 60s and even beyond to compete in such a demanding sport as track and field. But then Masters athletes were not average citizens—or if they began as such, they soon lost that designation when they started to compete.

I remember a conversation I overheard while in Victoria Station one afternoon during our trip. Because of traffic, it was easier to get to the Crystal Palace Sports Centre, where we were competing, by train than by taxi. While buying tickets, we stood in line dressed in our uniforms: red-white-and-blue sweat suits with "US Masters" on the back, striped running shoes, tote bags for our spikes, some of us carrying javelins and poles.

Behind me in line, a woman asked her husband, "Who are all these people in the athletic uniforms?"

Her husband shrugged, "They can't be runners. They're too old."

But, of course, we were not too old. That was the lesson taught us by David H. R. Pain. If Kenneth H. Cooper, M.D., is the Messiah of older athletes, Pain is their Moses. He led them out of the desert and into the green pastures of competition. He also correctly can be compared to Baron Pierre de Coubertin, the Frenchman who in 1896 almost single-handedly instituted the modern Olympic movement. David Pain, in similar fashion, was the singular force responsible for the outburst of athletic activity for oldsters, not only in Masters track and field but also (through the example set in that sport) in many other athletic areas.

But then David H. R. Pain is a singular individual. Lawyer, promoter, jogger, the man who brought the Batmobile to San Diego, he embodies the characteristics of Buddha and Daddy Warbucks. It is not merely that, with head as bald as a torpedo, he bears a superficial resemblance to both. It is more his philosophy of life.

First, in his quest for physical fitness, he seems to follow the principles of Buddhism, namely, that right living, correct thinking, and self-denial will enable the soul to reach a divine state of release from earthly sorrow and bodily pain. Second, as Daddy Warbucks might, he not only assumes a paternalistic attitude toward Masters track ("I can talk in terms of *my* program"), but he also does not hesitate to use force (a karate chop here, a lawsuit there) to bring the fruits of a better life to everybody.

"People who are nice never accomplish anything," states David Pain. "Anytime I've tried to be nice—on those rare occasions—somebody has spit on me. I learned as a lawyer you have to be willing to turn the screw. If not, you're in the wrong business."

David Pain never has hesitated to turn the screw. One time, he talked the San Diego Track Club into grabbing sponsorship of the profitable San Diego Indoor Games, causing the ousted meet promoter to label him a "bald pirate." On another occasion, the police arrested Pain for refusing to stop jogging on a municipal golf course. The arresting officer accused him of being a "ding-a-ling." In 1968, he organized the first national track and field championships for men in their 40s, earned $15,000 but ended suing his co-sponsor.

David Pain also feuds frequently with the press. A sports commentator acting as guest speaker at a San Diego Track Club banquet advised recruiting name athletes to club membership for their publicity value. Pain took the microphone afterward and retorted that anyone with a girth as ample as that of the commentator should not lecture on physical fitness. The commentator stormed out.

"Dave is brilliant as far as ideas," says Club member Bill Stock. "In diplomacy, he's zilch."

At a banquet for an amateur theatrics group, Pain found his conversation hindered by a rock band and asked them to play more softly. When they refused, he pulled the plug on their amplifier. On our tour to Europe in 1972, David and I had dinner following a cross-country meet in London with a number of competitors. The wife of one of the runners lit a cigarette. David told her, *please* put it out or leave the room!

"David is a bit feisty and just like a woodchuck," suggests San Diego Track Club member Bill Gookin. "Have you ever encountered a woodchuck? They're constantly busybodying. "

Ken Bernard, another SDTC member, nods his head: "Wherever there's a windmill. . . . ."

David Pain first turned to promotion in the early 1960s when his law firm had as a client Silver Gate Productions which organized the major custom car shows in Southern California. David became involved part-time in management of the company, thus his encounter with the Batmobile. At the height of the Batman craze, he contracted for the appearance of that car one weekend at the San Diego Custom Car Show. Unfortunately, by opening night Friday, the TV producers had fallen behind schedule and the Caped Crusader was still driving the Batmobile around a Hollywood set in his fight against the forces of evil.

"We displayed a notice that the Batmobile would not appear," recalls Pain. "We gave rain checks to anybody who complained. The next morning, we got confirmation that that car was on a flat-bed truck coming down from Hollywood. I got the bright idea to ask the Highway Patrol to let me know when the Batmobile reached the San Diego County line. Sure enough, around 10 I got word that the car had passed San Juan Capistrano. I immediately called the local disc jockeys and alerted them that the Batmobile was on its way, and as the car moved down the cost I kept getting more reports from the Highway Patrol who thought this was something of a lark. By the time we opened the doors at noon, there were 5000 people waiting. The fire marshalls finally had to close the doors because of the crowd."

While moonlighting as a custom car entrepreneur, Pain first encountered Al Franken, a sports promoter from the Los Angeles area. Franken sponsored many of the major track meets on the West Coast.

In 1964, Franken started a major outdoor meet in San Diego. The following year, he helped bring the National AAU Track and Field Championships to that city. He founded the San Diego Indoor Games. And in 1966, he allowed a San Diego attorney to talk him into allowing an event for runners over 40 in his outdoor meet.

The winning time in this first-ever "Masters mile" was slower than five minutes, and finishing more than a lap behind was gentleman jogger David H. R. Pain, the attorney who suggested the race. That Masters mile proved so successful that other meet promoters eventually copied it, and the avalanche of athletic competition for oldsters had begun. Although David Pain had no way of knowing it at the time, this avalanche would propel him into a position of leadership in the track world.

David Holland Rose Pain was born in Taplow, Buckinghamshire, England, on July 31, 1922. When he was five, his family moved to Windsor, Ontario, where his father worked on a Ford assembly line. They later settled in California because of David's health.

"Smog hadn't been invented yet," he comments, "and California was considered the ultimate place for people with consumption."

He started his own gardening business while attending North Hollywood High School, prospering to the point where he had four assistants caring for 22 yards. His senior year, he quit attending classes though stopping by daily for assignments. He would have graduated anyway had he not, early in 1941, enlisted in the Navy, which assigned him to the SS Washington, a luxury liner converted into a troop transport. On the day the Japanese attacked Pearl Harbor, Pain stood on the fantail of his ship off the South African coast and watched two torpedoes, fired by a lurking German submarine, narrowly miss blowing him to pieces.

The Washington sailed into Singapore under fog that prevented attacking Japanese airplanes from locating them and deposited the last reinforcements to that city, men whose later prison experiences inspired "The Bridge on the River Kwai." The ship next sailed to Port Said to pick up the famous "Rats of Tobruk," Australians who had spent two years defending that city against Rommel.

For three years, the SS Washington sailed the South Pacific, transporting fresh troops one direction, wounded the other, with David Pain more an observer than a participant in the shooting war. He finally applied for a commission through the Navy's V-12 program, attending college at Occidental and UCLA. Ninety days before earning his commission, he became eligible for discharge. Having previously dropped out of high school, he now dropped out of college, but nevertheless earned entry to the University of Southern California law school, where he met his future wife, Helen. He married Helen the following spring, honeymooned one weekend in San Diego and after graduation (his first) began practicing law in that city.

While establishing his own firm in Ocean Beach, he supplemented the family diet, and satisfied his own competitive urge, by surfing and spearfishing. "To this day I can go out and get my limit of abalone," he says. Helen learned how to make abalone pancakes, ab-waffles, ab-spaghetti and ab-burgers. Before the birth of the first of their four children, David got bored waiting in the hospital, and went out and caught a 15-pound lobster.

His law practice gradually expanded, and he added several partners, including Bob Pippen, who climbs mountains in his spare time. "He's a good lawyer in the courtroom," claims Pippen. "He's tenacious at digging out details." Pain is tenacious enough to have been threatened more than once for contempt of court. "The only thing Pain doesn't get chewed out about is long hair," says Pippen. Several years ago, Pain helped win the largest wrongful death verdict in San Diego County: $470,000 to the widow of a man killed in a commercial airline crash.

Too-frequent colds caused him to abandon surfing and skin-diving. He learned to fly. As a Los Angeles Rams season ticket holder, he often went to games by air. On one occasion, he found himself lost above the overcast in his twin-engine Beechcraft Bonanza with a failing battery, a non-functioning radio and his entire family. Fortunately, a hole appeared in the clouds, enabling him to land in El Cajon. The experience sobered him. He sold the plane, a decision made easier by the arrival in town of the San Diego Chargers.

He had begun playing handball and soon was serving as club handball commissioner, organizing competitive trips to Los Angeles and San Francisco.

"David can't be involved a little bit in anything," says friend Merle Hamilton. "When he goes in, it's with all four feet."

Pain fought with the club directors who refused to install different sidewalls despite their being ruined by paddleball players, quit the club and eventually dropped handball.

"First, I wasn't getting enough exercise," he says. "Second, it was too much of a hassle reserving courts and locating opponents. Third, I was getting home too late evenings. I started jogging mornings with my dog."

It did not take David Pain long to locate other joggers. One of them was Augie Escamilla, a student counselor at San Diego State, who worked out Sunday mornings with a group of older runners. For 12 years, Pain had spent Sunday mornings singing in the choir of the First Presbyterian Church.

"I enjoyed it," he says. "I don't think I missed a Sunday." But he dropped out of the choir to jog with Augie's group.

"For me to go to church on Sunday now is a total drag," admits Pain. "I'd rather go out and run for an hour. I have received more mental comfort from my running than from all the sermons I previously heard. There is something about being able to run on a beach or in a park in the quiet of nature that totally relieves you of the burdens of modern living. You develop an inner peace. You eliminate the turmoils and emotional stresses. I don't think runners make good church-goers, and it's for this very reason."

Running also caused Pain to abandon his seat on the 50-yard line at Charger games. "I'd rather be a participant than an observer," he says. Jogging, however, failed to satisfy Pain's natural competitive urge the way handball did. Handball players were much better organized competitively. They even had special categories for players over 40, as David Pain then was. The handball players adopted the term "Masters" to describe players in that category.

The US Handball Association added a Masters category to its national championships in 1952 in recognition of the fact that handball, because of the many bounces a ball can take off four surrounding walls, was a very difficult game to master. Once a player learns the angles, however, he often can play a control-pattern game, rarely having to move more than a step or two in either direction. Shrewd, mature players thus can play handball against faster, yet less experienced, players without excessive strain. Masters competition proved so popular that the US Handball Association later added Golden Masters (50 and over) and Super Masters (60 and over) divisions at its national championships.

David Pain reasoned logically: If such age divisions worked for handball, why wouldn't they be appropriate for track and field? He approached Al Franken, promoter of the San Diego outdoor meet, with this radical idea in 1966. Franken agreed to add a mile run for older runners.

It was an idea whose time had come. The Masters mile was reasonably popular with spectators but even more so with competitors. During the President Kennedy-inspired fitness boom in the early 1960s, older runners had been inspired to run in gyms, on tracks, along roads, in parks, with no way of measuring their achievement—and very little applause. Masters miles soon sprung up in other parts of the country. Two years after the first one in San Diego, David Pain took one step further and organized a full-event Masters track and field meet.

Competition at this first national championships for older runners was spotty and sometimes ludicrous. One runner appeared for the start of the 100-yard dash wearing house slippers with elastic bands to keep them on his feet. A shot putter sewed lace on his gym shorts. A smattering of Olympians—George Rhoden, Bob Richards, Bud Held—added class to early meets, but most participants had not competed in 20 years, and others never had tried the sport. They were reconstituted joggers: grandfather jocks.

As the Masters movement progressed, competition became tougher. Yet while improving in excellence, the Masters program did not lose its humanity: joggers still remained much a part of the scene. Division into five-year categories helped equalize competition. The Masters program also created an anomoly: men in their late 30s eagerly anticipated their 40th birthday.

Pain discovered he was not alone in being bored with being a spectator. He originally planned his veterans' tour of Europe in 1972 to attend the Olympic Games, with Masters track meets in England and Germany only diversions. When it seemed Olympic tickets at Munich might be scarce, he arranged alternate competitions in Helsinki, Stockholm and Copenhagen. Olympic tickets later became plentiful, but most tour members by then had decided they would rather run in Scandinavia than watch in Munich.

The early Masters meets in San Diego may not have been artistic successes, but incredibly they earned large sums of money—largely because of the promotional zeal of David H. R. Pain. His Silver Gate Productions once had sponsored a Christmas ice show to benefit the Arthritis Foundation, using a telephone soliciting company to sell $42,000 worth of tickets. Never one to abandon a good idea, Pain convinced the Arthritis Foundation to co-sponsor the first Masters meet. After all, what better publicity vehicle for such a charity than a bunch of old men running around a track? In the meet's first two years, this relationship earned the San Diego Track Club $5000 and $10,000 respectively.

"Lord knows what I would have made the third year if the club hadn't found out what I was doing," he says.

According to Ken Bernard, "It was the boilerhouse promotion outfit David had selling tickets: 50 solicitors in cubbyholes telephoning everybody in town. But people who bought tickets in January wouldn't come to the meet in July. This irritated many members."

They became further irritated when Pain had to sue the telephone soliciting company to recover the money. The San Diego Track Club quietly severed relations with its co-sponsors.

David Pain made several additional contributions to the meet, first getting the Amateur Athletic Union to recognize it as the national championships beginning in 1971, then getting the AAU to amend its rules to permit former professionals, assuming they were over 40, to compete in Masters competition. Former professional boxer Chuck Davey, who once fought Kid Gavilan for the world middleweight title, now competes as an amateur runner. Wes Santee, barred by the AAU in the mid-1950s for accepting money for running the mile, returned to competition. Many track coaches, also considered "professionals," found they could run again. Among them was Stanford and Olympic Coach Payton Jordan, who had been a world record-holder in his youth. He soon began setting world records for sprinters in their 50s.

Pain found other windmills to test with his lance. San Diego runners frequently took early morning workouts on private golf courses where they attracted little more than friendly waves from greenskeepers. On municipal golf courses, however, they often were abused by the management and chased from the fairways. Particularly, this was true at one public 36-hole course not far from Pain's La Jolla home: Torrey Pines, the site of the annual Andy Williams tournament.

To protest this situation, Pain appeared at a park board

meeting with Olympic champion Billy Mills. The board merely referred to committee their suggestion that joggers be allowed on public courses. Pain began to escalate the conflict, making certain he ran past the first tee, and the manager's office, on his morning run. On one occasion, he led a group of club runners through the grounds on a jog-in. Another time, a high school athletic breakfast at Torrey Pines provided the occasion for a mass workout on the fairways. Several times, the manager chased Pain in a golf cart and even tried to use a truck to run him down. Pain became adept at broken-field running.

Finally, one Sunday morning a policeman appeared, called by the management, to issue Pain a misdemeanor ticket for being on the golf course without having paid a greens fee. As he talked with the officer, Pain continued to jog in circles around the police car. The officer, dizzy, suggested they meet at the club parking lot.

"The officer was quite polite," remembers Pain. "He was only doing his job."

But then a police lieutenant arrived with another officer in a second squad car and began screaming at Pain, using obscenities, and calling him a "ding-a-ling." He ordered Pain spread-eagled and frisked. David's dog, Suzie, normally the most docile of animals, began barking loudly.

"Grab that dog!" snapped the lieutenant, and when one of the officers obeyed, Suzie bit him on the hand.

Pain was handcuffed, thrown into the back of the squad car, allowed to simmer in the hot sun, driven to the county jail, thrown into a cell with several drunks sleeping it off, and only several hours later was permitted to phone his wife.

"Hi, Helen," David began. "You'll never guess where I am."

Helen had no cash on hand and had to run to their oldest son Randy to borrow the money. Randy considered the request for a moment: "Now would Dad bail me out under similar circumstances?"

The arrest made the front page of the *San Diego Tribune* and was carried across the country by the wire services, not because of any sympathy for David H. R. Pain, gentleman jogger, but because Suzie had bitten the arresting officer. Later, Pain appeared in court where the presiding judge declared him not guilty of the misdemeanor of not having paid a greens fee since the course management could not sell joggers tickets, anyway. At a later meeting of the park board, the public golf courses were declared open to joggers as long as they did not interfere with the golfers. There is some sentiment among runners to have a brass plaque erected on the course commemorating the Battle of Torrey Pines.

Runners now train freely on public golf courses, but dogs still are banned. Pain usually runs mornings at a park near his office. Evenings after work, he runs on the beach at LaJolla Shores or at a nearby track. When he lived in LaJolla, he sometimes ran from his home to his office in Ocean Beach, a distance of eight miles. Before he installed a shower in his office, he would pause on the doorstep to squirt himself with a garden hose.

"He once had a meeting with two little old ladies," recalls Bob Pippen, "and all he had on was trunks. The average attorney doesn't do that."

In his law practice, Pain mostly has abandoned the general work to his partners while accepting only large cases that personally intrigue him. "I'm quite benign in my practice of law now," he admits.

He is less benign when it comes to athletics. After an operation in the spring of 1972 to remove a malignant mole on one leg, he returned to running too soon, ripping the stitches.

"All of us need releases of one form or another," he says. "For some it's alcohol or women. These character problems become apparent particularly after men get into their 40s. This is when men turn to booze, split up with their wives, become over-aggressive in business. As a lawyer, I run into these men all the time. They are totally amoral in their pursuit of the dollar, the making of the deal, the crunching under of their business opponents. These men are not necessarily interested in personal riches. Making money is merely a means of keeping score. They would just as soon put you in bankruptcy if they were playing for matches."

Pain cites the example of one wealthy businessman who briefly became active in Masters track, ran extremely well, won several races, but lost others and eventually quit competing possibly because he could not stand being second in anything. "He approached running by hysterically jetting from one race to another and standing on the starting line with a telephone in one hand, talking to his stockbrokers. He completely missed the point of running: using it to get rid of excess tension. Instead, it was making him more tense."

Pain also suggests that running can act as an aphrodisiac: "It can help men with their sex problems. Men who turn 40 frequently have real ego problems associated with sex and approaching inadequacy. In my law practice, I've handled hundreds of divorce cases. Very frequently, the woman's complaint was that their husband, even while very young, never got any exercise. He just let himself turn into a vegetable."

As the manager at Torrey Pines can attest, David H. R. Pain has not entirely sublimated his own aggressive tendencies in his running, but he is trying. "David always was bullheaded," admits Helen Pain. Pain's bullheadedness, however, has been the main reason why Masters track became established as a permanent fixture in the athletic world.

He refuses to claim all the credit: "It's not enough just to have a good idea," David told me recently when I visited him in San Diego. "It has to come along at the right time. But I do think Masters track is the most significant new thing to arise in a very old sport. People now can continue to participate even though their abilities have diminished. And this is the secret of Masters track, something that we must never lose sight of. It's the secret of age-group competition. We have had age-group competition for years with kids. Now we have all these old guys competing and having a wonderful time, because now they can win an event instead of being at the end of the pack.

"It's a chance to relive their youth. Either they missed athletics as a youth, like me, or they were in athletics and enjoyed it and this provides a chance to get back. There is a certain camaraderie in the sport, which is what gives me the motivation to try and stay fit. I don't think I'd train as hard if it were not for some upcoming races, like our trip to Sweden this summer, for example. (The second World Masters Track and Field Championships was scheduled for Goteborg, Sweden, in August 1977. The first World Championships in Toronto, Canada, in 1975 attracted 1300 competitors from 31 nations.) I probably wouldn't travel. I'd stay home or go backpacking somewhere on holiday. Now, I've become a world traveler as a result of the Masters program.

"The danger is that a sort of elitism is developing, particularly among people who only want to win, and see the program as merely a means of amassing more trophies and more medals. I think the American Medical Joggers and the National Jogging Association have the right approach, and that is to include everybody and not be so obsessed with individual performances. The only trouble is that track and field doesn't lend itself to not trying hard. You can't say, 'Well, fellows, let's run a mile on the track and not pay attention to who wins or your times.' That's not track and field.

"If you are going to have a program in track and field where you are measuring in hundredths of a second with electronic timing and measuring field performances in centimeters, people are going to look at those performances. It's inherent in the beast. I've been trying to run a five-minute mile since the day I got into Masters track. I've never succeeded. I got to 5:07 once, and that's my best. But five minutes is still my objective, and its people who are stimulated by such challenges who are led into the Masters program."

David H. R. Pain paused as he said that, perhaps realizing that he had become the Baron Pierre de Coubertin of the grandfather jocks. "You know," he finally said, "I get more compensation out of the Masters program because I can feel paternalistic about it. I can talk in terms of *my* program, and there's an ego trip involved in knowing you are somewhat instrumental in creating a program that's not only rewarding to yourself but rewarding to others."

7

Death of a Distance Runner

It was 7:30 on a Friday morning in July. A woman watering her lawn in the town of Pleasant Hill, a suburb of Oakland, Calif., glanced up in time to see the man in shorts and T-shirt stumble as he ran past. He fell to the sidewalk. She had seen him run past her house frequently, although she did not know his identity. At first, she thought he probably tripped. But he just lay there. When he failed to get up, she became worried and walked over to see what happened. He seemed to be unconscious.

"Are you all right?" asked the woman, but the downed runner failed to answer. The woman looked around for help and saw a policeman down the block writing out a parking ticket. She shouted for help.

The policeman came and glanced at the man on the pavement. "It looks like a heart attack," he mumbled and instructed the woman to go inside and call an ambulance. The policeman began giving the downed runner mouth-to-mouth resuscitation.

Several hours later, in a house a quarter-mile away, Bobbie

Shettler awoke and realized she had not heard her husband return from his morning run. "Jim!" she called, but there was no answer. It was then 10 a.m. She remembered him saying good-bye as he left that morning, but then she fell back to sleep. She had not been feeling well lately because of a cold.

Perhaps, she reasoned, he was taking a longer run than usual. Her husband, Jim Shettler, a 42-year-old long-distance runner, was training to race in a 26-mile, 385-yard race at Martins Beach, the Ocean-to-Bay Marathon, the following month.

But as Bobbie Shettler thought about it, she realized Jim had run 23 miles the day before. He and his training partner, Kent Guthrie, got lost running in the Oakland hills Thursday afternoon and stayed out three hours longer than planned. Jim joked about it when he returned, saying he covered 23 miles, farther than he'd ever run in his life. (Although he'd attempted several previous marathons, he never had finished one, usually because of his competitive nature; he ran too fast at the start.) Jim seemed tired from the long workout, but went off in good humor to teach his night classes at Diablo Valley College. He was head of the biology department.

When noon came and her husband still failed to return, Bobbie Shettler became seriously worried. She telephone a friend. "It's just not like Jim to go off and not call," she said.

She wondered what to do, then at 3 p.m. she saw two policemen approaching slowly up the walk. They seemed uncomfortable as she invited them in.

"I'm sorry, Mrs. Shettler," one of them finally announced, "your husband is dead."

Shocked, fighting back tears, she asked what happened. The policeman explained that her husband collapsed while running. They took him to the hospital emergency room, but it was too late.

"Which hospital?" she wanted to know.

"John Muir," the policeman replied.

"But we belong to the Kaiser plan," said Mrs. Shettler, realizing the moment the words left her mouth that was a silly thing to say. She was not thinking too clearly.

Bobbie Shettler kept hoping that somehow it was all a mistake. It could not be Jim. It must be some other runner who had died. Her hope collapsed when her husband was positively identified as the man lying lifeless on the examining table.

One of the policemen told her that her husband had been brought in off the ambulance, apparently dead on arrival. The physicians labored over him for 45 minutes, realizing that sometimes even a seemingly dead heart can be revived. They shocked him, attempted massage, injected heart-stimulating drugs, but all to no avail.

At 8:45 a.m. Friday, July 2, 1976, approximately an hour after stumbling during his morning run, Jim Shettler was pronounced officially dead. The delay in notifying his wife was because, clad only in running gear, carrying no wallet, there was no means of determining his identity. However, one of the policemen, who was enrolled in night school at Diablo Valley College thought he looked like one of the professors at that college. They made some calls, and a friend eventually showed up to make the identification.

"But what did he die of?" asked Bobbie Shettler, still stunned by the suddenness of what happened to Jim.

"A massive heart attack," announced the policeman.

She gasped, "I don't believe it!"

The shock waves from Jim Shettler's fall reverberated around the San Francisco Bay Area, one of the most active long-distance running areas in the United States. Each weekend throughout the year, there is at least one major road race near San Francisco and Oakland, with many minor ones as well. The Bay to Breakers Race, not the Boston Marathon, is America's largest running event. Winding 7.6 miles through the streets and across the hills of San Francisco, it attracts nearly 10,000 competitors each year. So great is the crush that officials long ago quit trying to record times and simply mounted a clock at the finish line. The Dipsea race, a 6.8-mile handicap event across Mt. Tamalpais, is one of America's toughest races. It also attracts several thousand entrants.

The two largest running publications—*Runner's World* and *Track & Field News*—are located in the area. Joggers, runners and racers can be seen everywhere, even striding through downtown San Francisco at the height of the rush hour. People no longer pay them much attention, they are so common.

When members of the Bay Area running community learned of Jim Shettler's death, they were stunned. "Not Jim?" they said, unwilling to believe it. "How did it happen?" they asked. Told his death came from a myocardial infarction, the classic heart attack, they shook their heads, unwilling to accept the verdict. "It can't be true." They seemed angry that anyone even dared suggest it.

Their cries of disbelief came because long-distance runners had come to believe that they could not die of heart attacks. Supposedly they possessed "immunity." Ask any runner why he runs, and the answers that come back are: it is fun, it makes him feel better, he enjoys the easy camaraderie at races. But tucked away in the back of his mind is the fact that running will make him live longer, that he can cheat Father Time.

Thomas Bassler, M.D., president of the American Medical Joggers Association, even has gone so far as to claim that if any individual trains for and completes a full-distance marathon (26 miles, 385 yards), and adopts what might be described as the Marathon Life Style (no smoking, low-fat diet, lots of exercise through running), he will be *immune* from a heart attack. Then what went wrong with Jim Shettler?

Shettler was not your average, off-and-on jogger; he was a champion runner. He was born Aug. 9, 1933 in San Francisco. As a teenager, he won the Dipsea. He set a record in the mile run at San Francisco State that lasted nine years. By 1960, he was one of America's fastest 3000-meter steeplechasers and might have made the Olympic team, had not an injury caused him to miss the trials. He retired from active competition after that but continued running three or four days a week. When he turned 40 in 1973, he became active in Masters running. At the world championships in Toronto in 1975, he placed fifth in the steeplechase. Only a few months before his death he won the National AAU Masters 25-Kilometer Championship. Then what went wrong with Jim Shettler?

After Shettler's death, Joe Henderson, editor of *Runner's World*, wrote an editorial in that publication: "We get reports on a half-dozen running related deaths each year. The runners who die usually fit a certain profile: coming back after decades of decadent living, less than a year into running, 10-20 pounds overweight, runs sporadically at short distances and too fast, had early symptoms of heart disease which might have been picked up by a stress test if he had taken one."

Jim Shettler failed to fit that profile. Two years prior to his death, he took a complete physical examination, including a stress test. He passed with no qualifications. Then what went wrong?

The death of Jim Shettler particularly bothered me because of many similarities in our lives, in our careers—something I realized only fully when I began checking his background. I ran in the 3000-meter steeplechase at the National AAU Championships in 1960 where Jim injured his foot on the water jump. I went on to the Olympic Trials; he did not.

Soon after turning 40, Jim traveled to Cleveland in 1973 for the National AAU Masters Cross-Country Championships. I won that race; he finished close behind. We ran together on the American team at the World Masters Championships in Toronto two years later, and Jim's 14th place helped us place second to Great Britain in the team race. I remember talking to him and his wife after the race. Three days later, Jim finished a short distance behind me when I won my gold medal in the steeplechase. He placed fifth, but he must have been disappointed. I don't recall seeing him after the race. The two of us were very close in ability and, I suspect, in temperament. I could easily visualize the finger that pointed at Jim Shettler shifting direction and pointing at me!

And at other runners. Running becomes a fixation, an addiction for us. If it came to a choice between several more years of full physical activity and many, many more years of the normal sedentary life lived by so-called average Americans, most runners would find themselves faced with a difficult choice.

It would be somewhat like the old comedy routine featuring Jack Benny. He was approached on the street by a robber, who accosts him and says, "Your money or your life!"

In the routine, there was a long, painful silence until finally the robber repeats the threat. *"I'm thinking about it!"* screams Benny.

I like to believe that if faced with a decision between my running and my life, I would choose the former. But you never know until the finger points your way.

Some months after Jim Shettler's death, I dined with David Pain, founder of the Masters movement for athletes 40 and over in track and field. He knew Jim Shettler well, liked him but wasted no time trying to rationalize his death.

"The Masters program has proved the fallibility of physical fitness," Pain admitted. "We would all like to think we are immortal, that we will live forever. But just being fit is no guarantee. We've had enough documented cases of superb athletes who had no history of heart disease kicking over."

One of David's close friends, Bill Hargus, recently died of an apparent heart attack. Hargus had a previous history of heart disease. He suffered a near-fatal myocardial infarction in the mid-1960s, recovered, and determined to rehabilitate himself by joining a physical activity clinic for heart patients run by Drs. Boyer and Cash at San Diego State University. He began walking, did light exercises, bicycled, jogged.

It was about the time the Masters movement got started in San Diego. During the course of the rehabilitative program, Bill Hargus got hooked on running, and completely changed his life style and that of his family. His wife Kathryn became a runner. His two daughters and son took up running, the son setting several age-group world records in the marathon. Bill ran the marathon faster than three hours at age 50.

"The family was very much into it," said David Pain.

Then one night Bill Hargus went to sleep and failed to wake up. "Bill was on borrowed time and he knew it," explained David. "Running gave him an additional 10 years of good life, and when he went, he died in his sleep, which is about the best way I know of going."

About the same time, Don Palmer, a man in his 40s who ran the quarter-mile for the Corona del Mar track team, a club consisting mostly of older runners, stopped off at a shopping center following a vigorous workout. They found his body next to his car the next morning. He was dead of an apparent heart attack.

And in Vancouver, British Columbia, Dr. Leslie Truelove, who had taken up running six years earlier at age 47 to increase his fitness, came to the 21-mile mark during the Lion's Gate International Marathon and collapsed. He had run only three miles a day until a year previous, when he doubled his mileage in an attempt to finish a marathon. An autopsy later indicated that one of his arteries burst.

Dr. Truelove may have entered the marathon spurred by the challenge, or he might have been on a quest for immortality, following the theory that a marathon a year keeps the coroner away, the hypothesis presented by Dr. Thomas Bassler of the American Medical Joggers Association, who believes that the ability to finish a marathon confers immunity to heart attack on those who do so. Dr. Bassler not only believes this, he has not hesitated to publicize his beliefs, which have been misinterpreted to mean that if you rush out and finish a marathon you're cardiac-proof for life. Of course, Dr. Truelove never got to the finish line.

Such cases caused many in the medical profession to become concerned over the interpretation of Dr. Bassler's remarks, and several members of the American Medical Joggers Association cautioned him that in describing his theories of immunity he should make it perfectly clear he was speaking as an individual, not as their president.

Seymour Dayton, M.D., a Los Angeles physician, responded to an article by Dr. Bassler in the *New England Journal of Medicine* by writing angrily, "Until somebody publishes analyzable data, I hope we could enjoy a moratorium on public assertions that marathon running prevents coronary heart disease."

Joan Ullyot, M.D., author of the book *Women's Running*, a former pathologist who now works at the Institute of Health Research at the Pacific Medical Center, and a sub-three-hour marathoner at age 36, does not entirely accept Dr. Bassler's immunity theories. But she refuses to concede that running—or any other form of exercise—is bad for your health. She notes that when a jogger dies, it makes headlines simply because it is so unusual.

"Any physician knows that a much, much higher percentage of people die of heart attacks while having sexual intercourse or straining on the toilet," she states. "You rarely read about those causes in the obituary columns."

Yet, while researching this book, it was difficult to overlook the fact that people do die while participating in one form or another of physical exercise, presumably cheated in their bid for immortality. Chuck Sheftel, a racquetball instructor at the Mid-Town

Court House in Chicago, cited two cases. He knew of one individual who, to lose weight, played racquetball while clad in a rubber suit weight at one of the Court House chain of clubs. The strain was too much; he died of a heart attack. He knew of another individual who went into the sauna after a strenuous game of tennis at another club and failed to come out alive. The winner of a national 45-year-old division tennis championship recently needed a coronary bypass because of a heart condition.

When I was preparing the earlier chapter in this book on coronary bypass, Dr. Marlin Silver told me, "In the last two months, I've operated on five patients who have had cardiac arrests in various stages of tennis, racquetball or jogging. Three of the five were good friends. They were men either 40- or 50-plus, interested in physical conditioning and obviously almost killed themselves doing it."

He added, "I understand that somebody died at Sky Harbor Court Club last week playing racquetball. I learned that when I was playing the other night, but I fully expected to hear something like that for the past year. It's a very strenuous activity for the average person to start without preparation."

While interviewing David L. Costill, Ph.D., director of the Human Performance Laboratory at Ball State University, he mentioned two deaths at the YMCA in Muncie, Ind. These were individuals who had failed to undertake physical examinations before starting exercise. Physiologist Dr. Alan Claremont, visiting Costill at that time, described a man, determined to begin a long-postponed exercise program, who appeared at his laboratory at the University of Wisconsin to take a stress test. The man decided against it on discovering the price would be $75.

"He went to a nearby gym," explained Claremont, "did six chin-ups, then fell from the bar. Physicians from our laboratory arrived within 19 seconds yet failed to save him."

Claremont added, "Few insurance companies yet seem willing to reimburse customers who take stress tests, although they sometimes pay more in early death benefits."

People also die while taking stress tests, although in relatively few numbers. The death rate once was one in 10,000, claims William Carlyon, M.D., of the American Medical Association. It is now one in 15,000.

"The risk is slight," says Dr. Carlyon, "except for that one person. It's 100% for him."

I have heard of fewer problems among competitive swimmers, although several years ago the 50-year-old former records chairman for the Masters swim program emerged from the swimming pool following a strenuous workout, walked into the locker room and died.

"A lot of people who participate in Masters programs are non-athletes," cautions Dr. David Costill. "When they get to be 35, they start jogging, and before you know it they become competitive and start running a few races. The danger is that some people may have cardiovascular problems without realizing it. They can exercise, but probably they should not compete. The spirit of competition may cause them to push themselves too far."

When I interviewed Herman K. Hellerstein, M.D., he admitted that he felt jogging had been oversold by individuals such as *Aerobics* author, Kenneth H. Cooper, M.D. "People seem preoccupied with jogging," stated Dr. Hellerstein, "but running does not do enough to improve arm mobility." He took a particularly dim view of competitive distance races, saying, "I dislike mass running. The whole concept of immunity is a myth. Marathon running is an unnecessary display of talent."

Dr. Hellerstein is an area chairman for the American Heart Association, which takes an equally conservative approach toward jogging as a means of fitness. "They almost don't recommend it," said William Carlyon, M.D., of the American Medical Association. "They are concerned about the middle-aged guy who decides to get out and run and overdoes it. They think the hazards are greater than the benefits. They prefer walking."

Dr. Carlyon, who is a runner, adds, "I don't agree with them."

In nearly 30 years of competition, during which I have competed in hundreds of races from 100 yards to the marathon, sometimes in fields of thousands, I only recall being in one race where a runner died. That was at the National AAU Track and Field championships in St. Louis in 1954, on a day when the temperature soared above 100. It was still 98 degrees when we began the 10,000 meters in the early evening.

During the last few miles, I became locked in a battle for fourth place with Austin Scott of the New York Pioneer Club. I passed him. He passed me. I passed him again. He seemed to be wheezing badly, but he pulled away in the last few laps to finish ahead of me—then collapsed.

I became sick and later threw up in a potted palm back at the hotel. I never did that at a race before or since, but Austin Scott was even sicker. A week later, I learned he died in the hospital, never having regained consciousness. A complication in his case, newspaper reports stated, was a recent hepatitis infection. He should not have been running.

None of use should have been running in that heat, but competition sometimes drives athletes to extend their abilities. Some years later, I ran another race in 96-degree heat, the Olympic Marathon Trial in Yonkers, N.Y., which the Olympic Committee scheduled to begin at high noon. I was running in second place at about 17 miles when I began to hear ringing in my ears. I slowed my pace and the ringing went away; I sped up and the ringing came back. I dropped out of the race and Norm Higgins, who moved into second when he passed me, later went straight when the road turned left and he ran into a wall. He spent one week in the hospital. You hear of race drivers failing to make turns and crashing, but Norm was traveling only 10 miles per hour.

But Norm, Austin and I were young runners in our 20s and 30s when felled under stress. The dangers of death increase as men in their 40s, 50s and 60s continue to compete—or begin to compete. In Stockholm, Sweden in 1972, I was dressing to run a 1500-meter race in a veterans' track meet when David Pain came into our dressing room and announced that Martti Laitinen, a man in his 60s who was part of our tour group, collapsed in the park during the walking race that preceded the track meet.

"It looks like a heart attack," David admitted. "His face looked very grey. Martti could talk but could not see. They rushed him to the hospital."

One of the fears of those involved with veterans' running was that, should someone die during competition, others would look upon this as proof that athletics for middle-aged men was unsafe. A sprinter suffered a heart attack the previous year at a meet in San Diego, but recovered. He never raced again.

When I learned of Martti's plight, I felt sorrow, but I also envied him. We had sat near each other on the bus taking us to our hotel in Helsinki, Finland, for another track meet a few days earlier. He was laughing, making jokes in Finnish with a drunk who got on our tour bus by mistake. Martti had been born in Finland and left his native land in 1931 while still in his 20s. The track tour was an excuse for him to return and visit his family, including his sister whom he had not seen in 41 years. It had been a pleasant family reunion, then came his heart attack two days later.

If I had to choose my end, I would be stricken down while running through the piney forest. But it did not work entirely that way with Martti. He spent several weeks in the hospital in Sweden, recovered and returned home to Seattle. He admitted afterwards on the telephone to David Pain that he had trained insufficiently for his event. Soon afterwards, he died.

The main danger older athletes must face is the inability of arteries clogged with atherosclerotic deposits to supply the heart muscles with sufficient oxygen-containing blood. Deprived of oxygen, the heart may stop, the same way an automobile engine deprived of gasoline will stop.

In testing more than 500 middle-aged men at the Human Performance Laboratory, Dr. David Costill discovered that one out of 10 had oxygen deficiencies because of a poor cardiovascular system. That person might be able to stand the stress of gradual training but not the extreme stress of intense competition.

The curve goes up dramatically with age. Costill never found a man over 65, including competitive athletes, who did not show inadequate oxygen supply to the heart muscles during a maximum stress test. He feels the greatest risk is to people who do not get involved in athletics until middle age:

"The critical years in terms of cardiovascular disease are between 25 and 35. That's the era of a man's life, and women too, when they pay the least attention to their physical health. A man will be busy with his job and family, and never pay any attention to his endurance ability. He will let himself deteriorate. Once you build up atherosclerotic deposits in your system, you rarely get rid of it—even by exercise. At best, you can stop the build-up of more deposits, or hope that by being better trained you will have more strength to survive a heart attack should it occur."

Perhaps that was what motivated Henry Jordan, a defensive tackle from the Green Bay Packers of the Lombardi era, who was jogging in a Milwaukee gym in February 1977 as part of a fitness program. He fell dead of a heart attack.

I can understand the death of a former football player, knowing their life style, the rich steaks, plates of scrambled eggs and bacon, pitchers of milk that they wolf down in order to maintain the size necessary to play in the National Football League. Once retired from their sport, with no coach threatening fines for reporting overweight, they would seem to be likely candidates for heart attacks.

But how do you explain the death of someone with a Marathon Life Style? How do you explain Jim Shettler?

That question bothered Jim's wife, Bobbie, who knew the sudden paranoia that must be gripping the running community in the Bay Area. Jim's friends now saw the finger of fate pointed at them.

"I lived with a runner for 20 years," comments Bobbie Shettler. "I know what they're like."

The day after Jim's death, she talked with Kent Guthrie, Jim's frequent training partner, who had gone with him on the 23-mile workout the day before his death. They decided to ask a physician familiar with running to re-examine the coroner's report.

"Jim loved running," she told Kent. "He wouldn't want the sport hurt by his death."

"I feel the same way," Kent Guthrie agreed.

The physician they chose was Joan Ullyot, M.D., herself a runner and a former pathologist. A suddenly awakened interest in sports at the age of 30 caused Joan to shift from pathology to sports medicine so she could prevent people from dying rather than examining them after their death. Kent contacted Joan, who agreed to determine the exact cause of Jim Shettler's death.

Dr. Ullyot first called the coroner's office, to which Jim Shettler's body had been taken, and asked to speak with the pathologist who performed the autopsy. He was not present, so Dr. Ullyot asked the nurse who answered the telephone to read her report. It indicated that Jim Shettler died of a massive myocardial infarction, caused by extensive coronary atherosclerosis and cardiomeggaly.

"He had an enlarged heart," explained the nurse.

"Of course, he had a large heart," said Dr. Ullyot. "He was a distance runner."

"Oh," said the nurse. "We didn't know that."

Dr. Ullyot asked what else they checked: "Did he have a ruptured aorta? Could there have been a hemorrhage in the brain? Did you check the adrenals? Was there anything else that could have caused him to fall like that?"

The nurse admitted, no. "The doctor saw the enlarged heart," she said, "and took it from there."

Joan Ullyot sighed. She knew her task would not be simple.

Later, Dr. Ullyot visited the coroner's office for a personal examination of the heart. She discovered that the coroner had been mistaken in his diagnosis of myocardial infarction. There was no sign of such a condition in Jim's heart muscle.

What she did discover was an occlusion of the left anterior coronary artery, one of the three principal arteries supplying blood to the heart muscle and, particularly, to the conduction system of the left ventricle. This particular artery was 90% obstructed, "perhaps totally so," Dr. Ullyot said later.

Apparently because of this blockage, the oxygen supply into one particular piece of conductive tissue, which regulates the beat of the heart, was shut off. The heart apparently went into what physicians refer to as an arrythmia. In automotive terms, it is less like the supply of gasoline being shut off (as in a myocardial infarction), but more like a misfunctioning of the electrical system. For Jim Shettler, it was as though someone suddenly had plucked the rotor from his distributor.

Such an arrythmia may not necessarily prove fatal. "We've seen similar patterns when we put monitors on world-class runners," Joan Ullyot explained to me when we talked one morning in Gainesville, Fla. The night before, we had spoken before a group of 400 at a running clinic. Within a few hours, we would be running in a 10-mile race.

"They sometimes have brief electrical disturbances," Joan continued. "They can have premature ventricular beats, even two or three of them in a row, and their hearts, being healthy and well supplied with oxygen, just resume their normal conductive patterns. A healthy heart is no more damaged by scattered, or even coupled, irregular beats than one beating regularly. A heart with coronary artery disease, however, is more vulnerable."

But how healthy was Jim Shettler's heart? Joan Ullyot replied, "There was one segment, about one centimeter long, narrowed by accumulated cholesterol deposits. Apart from that, his arteries were generally free of atherosclerosis, and the heart muscle itself appeared strong and free of any evidence of poor oxygen supply, such as old scars. The most likely cause of death then was an arrythmia—disturbance of the heart rhythm—resulting from coronary artery disease which interfered with blood flow to the conductive tissue."

Joan paused, then summarized her finding: "Definitely you can say that Jim's heart was originally fine, except he had coronary artery disease. Very localized. Minimal. But very fatal."

But there had to be reasons why even this could occur in a seemingly healthy runner. Only when you dig very carefully into Jim Shettler's past do you uncover clues as to the cause of his death. His father suffered a near-fatal infarction while still in his 30s, surviving to his 70s but eventually succumbing of a heart attack as did his father, Jim's grandfather. Several of Jim's uncles died of heart attacks. In fact, a total of six members of Jim's immediate family had heart disease. It was a genetic flaw in the Shettler family, like hemophilia in the Hapsburg kings. To escape this fate was one reason that prompted Jim Shettler to continue running.

And there was another clue: At age 14, Jim had arrythmic problems with his heart. These disappeared after a year and seemed to be no reason for him not to indulge in physical activity.

"You can't do much about heredity," Joan Ullyot explained. "It is one of the major reasons for heart attacks: strong family history of heart disease, smoking, overweight, stress, high blood pressure, high cholesterol. All these things are risk factors, and, of course, he eliminated almost all of them except family history."

Other factors may have contributed to his eventual death, one of them stress. Jim Shettler was extremely active: a painter, a wine-maker, a sailor. He was interested in ecology, and belonged to the Sierra Club and Audubon Society. He served as campaign manager for the first woman elected to the Pleasant Hill city council. During the previous year, he was appointed chairman of the biology department at Diablo Valley College. It was a position he did not relish.

"Jim was a teacher, not an administrator," comments his wife Bobbie. There was considerable conflict at the time because of collective bargaining negotiations.

Meyer Friedman, M.D., considers stress a major factor in causing heart attacks and suspects that it perhaps triggers changes in the body that could, in some people—those he classifies as Type A individuals—increase the amount of cholesterol in their blood stream. Or perhaps stress causes them to change their habits—such as eating more fat-laden foods, smoke more cigarettes, drink more alcohol, all forms of compensation—which could cause a buildup of atherosclerotic deposits.

Jim Shettler was extremely competitive. Most successful competitive racers fit the Type A pattern much more than fitness joggers. We are concerned with times. Jim pushed himself in practice so he could be a front-runner, win races, achieve fast times. He started several marathon races, but failed to finish mainly because of his competitive nature.

"He would try to run a time near 2:30," explained Joan Ullyot. "When he got out past 20 miles, started to fade and saw he would finish slower than 2:50, he simply quit."

The failure to finish a marathon bothered Jim Shettler, so he increased his training, averaging 10 miles a day, 70 miles a week, to see if he could get to the finish line in respectable time. The American Masters record in the marathon was only 2:28:27. Jim knew, and others knew, that it probably was well within his capabilities if he just trained for it and had a good day. He already was looking beyond the race in August to the national Masters race in Honolulu in December which would be on a flat course, in good weather, making a record highly possible.

In the last two weeks before his death, he suddenly began feeling tired. His wife Bobbie noticed this. "He looked tired," she said, but thought her husband merely was showing the classic symptoms of overtraining. He appeared extremely fatigued following his long 23-mile run with Kent Guthrie on Thursday, but he rested, ate a normal dinner and left to teach his classes at night school from 7-10. He came home and soon after went to bed.

Then Friday morning he rose to go for that morning run.

Was Jim Shettler's death preventable? Joan Ullyot, M.D., answered: "It was a freaky think. If his condition had been detected early, which was unlikely, I might have told him not to race, but he was not racing at the time he had the disturbance."

Could better, or more prompt, treatment have revived him? Joan Ullyot shook her head: "It's fate. Presumably, if he had fallen right in the emergency room of the hospital he might have survived. They can revive a person with arrythmia, whose heart is fibrillating, by use of cardio-pulmonary resuscitation. Had he survived, at that point they would have recommended a coronary bypass, because by then the occlusion of his artery would have been symptomatic.

His wife said Jim was scheduled to have a multi-phasic physical only a few weeks after his death. Would that have warned him? Dr. Ullyot said, "I don't think his condition could have been diagnosed even by a stress test, because his heart was so strong it would have masked this little area of occlusion. If he had no pain, there would have been no reason to do the operation. Unless people have symptoms, doctors won't operate on them, or the people don't want the operation."

She felt, judging from the generally healthy condition of Jim's coronary arteries, running probably prolonged his life. "As for the actual circumstances of Jim's death," she concluded, "a fatal arrythmia could have occurred at any time—while sleeping or watching TV or walking. Running was not the cause of death."

Yet Jim Shettler was a well-conditioned runner whose heart failed him. After talking to Joan, I called Tom Bassler, M.D., whose well-publicized views that marathoners never die of heart attacks seemed to be disproved. "Are you still saying 'never'?" I asked him.

"I'm still saying never," Dr. Bassler replied calmly. He explained he appeared at a medical clinic connected with the New York Marathon in October 1976. Physicians from 13 countries appeared, many of them to challenge him. One who appeared to do battle was Tim Noakes, M.D., of South Africa, who brought with him examples of five individuals who all completed marathons and all had heart attacks. One of them, a 2:33 marathoner, died.

"Bassler's widely publicized views have dangerous clinical

application and have for all practical purposes been disproved," Dr. Noakes told a reporter from *Medical News* before the meeting.

But Dr. Bassler defended his views, stating his careful qualification that myocardial infarction must be proved by autopsy. "Everybody scoured their cases and brought them all to New York," he commented later, "and it was just a total failure. The kind of cases they brought were of not only persons who did not have autopsies, but nobody knew anything about them. There would be a 38-year-old marathoner, and he was dead, and we had no information at all, but somebody decided it had to be a heart attack."

At the same conference, Dr. Noakes eventually admitted that he failed to disproved Dr. Bassler's hypothesis: "We still haven't got a dead marathoner with coronary artery atherosclerosis proved by pathology."

Dr. Bassler added, "When I learn of an autopsy report that says something like heart disease, or stroke, or certain types of cancer that killed a runner over 40, I am skeptical. If it's a marathoner, I look for the types of death you would expect in a teenager. We've been doing that for 10 years and never have been disappointed."

But what about someone like Bill Hargus, the marathoner with the history of heart disease who died in his sleep? Dr. Bassler said, "He may have died of a brain tumor. He had gone through a personality change in the previous few months. He had headaches, yet they failed to check the brain in autopsy."

And Dr. Truelove, who died in the marathon in British Cclumbia? "He never got to the finish line. He was trying to do so but he collapsed before succeeding."

And Jim Shettler? "It could have been a potassium death. He might have lowered his potassium level by overtraining the day before, triggering the arrythmia. And he never finished a marathon. These cases start out being marathoners with heart attacks, and they end up being non-marathoners."

Joan Ullyot concedes that Jim Shettler never finished a marathon, thus his cause falls outside Dr. Bassler's very narrow definition of immunity from heart attack for anyone who finished a marathon and continues to live a Marathon Life Style. She feels, however, that by demanding proof of heart damage by autopsy

Dr. Bassler has raised a qualifying wall that may be too difficult to scale. A sudden death from a heart attack, provided death came instantaneously, might not even damage the heart muscle, so it would be undetectable on autopsy. Joan insists also that Jim Shettler, despite never finishing a marathon, *could* have finished one if that were his only goal and that his arrythmia, though not a myocardial infarction, nevertheless was a form of heart attack.

Paul Milvy, Ph.D., a researcher at Mt. Sinai School of Medicine in New York, also says that the Marathon Life Style, not the actual running of full-distance marathons, may be the most important factor in granting so-called immunity. He states, "The overwhelming majority of marathoners are thin, do not smoke, drink sparingly and minimize their consumption of meat, and perhaps the style of living required of long-distance running may reduce risk factors for coronary atherosclerosis—rather than the running itself."

Dr. Bassler concedes this may be true, but nevertheless says, "We're still standing firm. We're seeing heart patients, seemingly hopeless ones, turning into marathon runners, and you can't tell them from the others in the race. They're usually doing it against their doctor's advice. They're the ones who are teaching the doctors."

Despite disagreeing with Tom Bassler on technicalities, Joan Ullyot nevertheless agrees with him on a much broader point: "It is silly to condemn running because somebody happens to die, and he was a runner. I would rather condemn TV-watching. But it's quite clear that there is no such thing as absolute protection, and anyone who is counting on absolute protection from heart disease because they run the marathon is fooling himself."

When I spoke to Joan Ullyot in Gainesville, she also told me a story about Ben Hirsch, a man in his 70s who coincidentally I had met at a party in San Francisco only the month before. Ben went to the Cooper Clinic for a physical examination and learned he had an irregularity in his heartbeat, one not dissimilar to what killed Jim Shettler. The irregularity was more apparent during rests; his heartbeat smoothed out when he took his stress test.

Nevertheless, one of the physicians recommended that Ben not run more than a half-hour, or about three miles, a day—probably sound advice, although Joan wryly commented that since Ben's heart beat better during exercise, he might be safer exercising all the time and resting only a half-hour.

Ben Hirsch followed the advice, but eventually got inspired by the camaraderie of the Dolphin-South End Club in San Francisco and soon progressed to running marathons. He remembered the physician's advice, however, and one day after a workout expressed to another runner a fear that he might die while running. That individual, Walt Stack, a man in his late 60s, in addition to running daily also swims an hour before dawn in the local waters of San Francisco Bay.

Stack told him, "Don't worry. The way I look at it, there is only one better way to go." Ben Hirsch thought about it, and decided that the advice was sound. He continued to run without worry. Walt Stack's better way to go, of course, was during sexual intercourse—or, as he more bluntly expressed it, "in the saddle."

The previous summer, Walt Stack was running in the Pike's Peak Marathon, a race to the summit of that 14,110-foot mountain in Colorado. Stack does not run as much as he trots, usually at the same pace, no matter the distance or difficulty of the event. They have a saying at the Dolphin-South End Club that if you pushed Walt Stack out of an airplane, he still would fall at the rate of eight minutes per mile.

Nearing the summit of Pike's Peak, Stack found himself in the company of a woman runner. They came to a monument to an 88-year-old woman who ascended Pike's Peak 15 times and died in her final attempt.

Walt was moved by the moment. "What could be better than to die climbing Pike's Peak," he commented. "That's almost as good as dying in the saddle."

"Yes, you're right," the woman replied.

The two continued up the mountain together and, despite the thin air, Walt Stack continued to expand upon his views about dying in the saddle. He considered the woman very broad-minded because she kept nodding and agreeing with him until they got to the summit.

Then she turned to Stack and said, "Walt, I just can't understand why you are so concerned about dying on horseback."

Whether you accept Walt Stack's set of priorities, some ways of dying are superior to others. I thought of Jim Shettler with his family history of heart attacks—his father dead of coronary artery disease, his grandfather dead of coronary artery disease, four other close relatives dead of coronary artery disease—and it was obvious that he had lived life as though atop a ticking time bomb. Of course, he had not expected it to explode as fast as it did.

I also thought of my own father, dead of a heart attack at age 69. A number of sudden stresses at work and at home seemed to push him over the edge. It took him three days to go after his first and only heart attack. He was propped up in a hospital bed, the green line on the electrocadiograph monitor representing his heart bouncing irregularly, tubes stuck in his nose, lines into his arms, and oxygen being forced through a mask into his lungs and through them into arteries clogged through disuse.

My father was physically inactive. He went to work, he came home, he went to work. With all the tubes and lines and masks, he could not communicate verbally, but his eyes pleaded for help. Then, while I was waiting in the reception room, one of the nurses came out and told me it was too late for help. When I re-entered my father's room, the green line on the scope that previously bounced irregularly was now straight.

I wondered then, as I looked at my dead father, if that would some day be my fate—10 years, 20 years, 30 years in the future. My father did not want to die in a hospital bed, nor do I. And as I think now of Jim Shettler, I cannot help but almost envy him.

"Jim knew about his family's history of heart problems," his wife Bobbie told me when we talked. "Jim said, 'That's eventually what's going to get me,' but he never thought it would get him until he was at least 80 or 90 years old. Running was kind of his life insurance. That's the way he looked upon it, as well as his life style and his recreational activity. And I think he liked the stimulation of competition, too.

"But he also looked upon it as a way to stay fit and to live a long and healthy life. He had the idea that it kept him feeling good. It wasn't the quantity, it was the quality of life that interested him. He always felt that when he was in peak shape, he enjoyed life more and could do more. And I like to think about that, because if anybody crammed a lot into 42 years, Jim Shettler did. He didn't waste a minute."

8
What Is Your True Athletic Potential?

Ken Young, director of the National Running Data Center in Tucson, Ariz., examined the age records of events from 100 meters to the marathon at my request to develop a series of charts by which older athletes could compare their performances with those of younger athletes. Young was surprised to find very little difference in the decline between sprint and endurance activities.

"This suggests that the decline is similar for all functions pertinent to athletic endeavor," he commented. Ever the statistician, Young speculated that if he had a set of similar data from other, unrelated activities he might be able to verify this hypothesis.

It has only been recently that older athletes have had the opportunity to compete in sports such as track and field and swimming. The Masters movement is now worldwide. But how good is the 10.7 time for 100 meters run by Thane Baker at age 41? How good is the 4:47.1 mile run by George Sheehan, M.D., at age 50? How good is the 2:58:40 marathon run by John A. Kelly at age 61? Ken Young's tables now permit us to make some guesses.

The answer, in the case of each of these fine athletes, is that if Thane Baker, George Sheehan and John A. Kelly had run their races at the ages that statisticians tell us are optimal for best performances in their events, they would have run 9.83, 4:09.6 and 2:18:46, respectively.

Anyone using Ken Young's charts can make a similar determination of the value of his or her performances. (Although Ken found very little difference in the decline between the 100-meter dash and the marathon, the percentage values differ because of differing "optimum ages." The process by which you determine your true athletic potential is relatively simple, although it helps to own a battery-powered pocket calculator, and to have a pencil and paper handy. Here is how it works:

Take, for example, Thane Baker's time of 10.7 seconds for 100 meters at age 41. By consulting the following tables, you can determine that the theoretical decline for a sprinter at that age at that distance made him 8.8% slower than a young sprinter. Divide the time of 10.7 seconds by 1.088, and you obtain a theoretical time of 9.83 seconds, a mark statistically superior to the actual world record of 9.95 set by Jim Hines at the Olympics in Mexico City in 1968. (Baker's race, however, was hand-timed in tenths of a second, which under current standards would invalidate it for world records which now must be timed electronically in hundredths for IAAF approval.)

A similar assessment can be made on Dr. Sheehan's time of 4:47.1 for the mile at age 50. The tables say he has declined an estimated 15%. In analyzing times over 60 seconds, however, you must remember to convert minutes into seconds. Sheehan's time thus becomes 287.1 seconds, divided by 1.15, which equals 249.65. His mile time is the equivalent of 4:09.6 for a young runner, a mark he can be proud of although it seemingly does not match Thane Baker's world record conversion. While competing for Manhattan College, Sheehan actually ran 4:17 at age 21. Busy with medical studies, he did not remain in competition by his theoretical peak age of 25.

John A. Kelly's marathon of 2:58:40 at age 61 also can be analyzed. First, the time in hours must be converted into time in minutes, or 178:40. then the time in minutes must be converted into time in seconds, or 10,720. Divide this time by the age 61

Equivalent Performance

Age	100 Meters	Mile	Marathon	
23	10.0 11.0			
24	10.0 11.0	4:00 5:00		
25	10.1 11.1	4:01 5:01		
26	10.1 11.1	4:01 5:01		
27	10.1 11.1	4:01 5:02		
28	10.1 11.1	4:01 5:02		
29	10.2 11.2	4:02 5:03	2:30:00	3:00:00
30	10.2 11.2	4:03 5:03	2:30:09	3:00:11
31	10.2 11.3	4:03 5:04	2:30:27	3:00:32
32	10.3 11.3	4:04 5:05	2:30:45	3:00:54
33	10.3 11.4	4:05 5:06	2:31:03	3:01:16
34	10.4 11.4	4:06 5:07	2:31:30	3:01:48
35	10.5 11.5	4:07 5:09	2:31:57	3:20:20
36	10.5 11.6	4:09 5:11	2:32:51	3:03:25
37	10.6 11.7	4:10 5:13	2:33:36	3:04:19
38	10.7 11.7	4:12 5:14	2:34:30	3:05:24
39	10.7 11.8	4:13 5:17	2:35:33	3:06:40
40	10.8 11.9	4:15 5:19	2:36:45	3:08:06
41	10.9 12.0	4:17 5:21	2:37:57	3:09:32
42	11.0 12.1	4:19 5:24	2:39:18	3:11:10
43	11.0 12.1	4:21 5:26	2:40:39	3:12:47
44	11.1 12.2	4:23 5:29	2:42:00	3:14:24
45	11.2 12.3	4:25 5:33	2:43:30	3:16:12
46	11.3 12.4	4:27 5:34	2:45:09	3:19:11
47	11.3 12.5	4:29 5:37	2:46:39	3:19:59
48	11.4 12.6	4:31 5:39	2:48:18	3:21:58
49	11.5 12.7	4:34 5:42	2:49:57	3:23:56

Age	100 Meters	Mile	Marathon
50	11.6 12.8	4:37 5:46	2:51:45 3:26:06
51	11.7 12.9	4:39 5:49	2:53:33 3:28:16
52	11.8 13.0	4:42 5:53	2:55:30 3:30:36
53	11.9 13.1	4:45 5:56	2:57:27 3:32:58
54	12.1 13.3	4:48 6:00	2:59:24 3:35:17
55	12.2 13.4	4:51 6:04	3:01:21 3:37:37
56	12.3 13.6	4:55 6:08	3:03:18 3:39:58
57	12.5 13.7	4:58 6:12	3:05:15 3:42:18
58	12.6 13.8	5:01 6:16	3:07:12 3:44:38
59	12.7 14.0	5:04 6:20	3:09:09 3:46:59
60	12.9 14.1	5:07 6:24	3:11:15 3:49:30
61	13.0 14.3	5:11 6:28	3:13:21 3:52:01
62	13.1 14.5	5:14 6:32	3:15:27 3:54:32
63	13.3 14.6	5:18 6:37	3:17:42 3:57:14
64	13.4 14.8	5:21 6:41	3:19:57 3:59:56
65	13.6 14.9	5:25 6:46	3:22:12 4:02:38
66	13.7 15.1	5:28 6:50	3:24:27 4:05:20
67	13.9 15.3	5:32 6:55	3:26:51 4:08:13
68	14.0 15.4	5:36 6:59	3:29:06 4:10:55
69	14.2 15.6	5:39 7:04	3:31:30 4:13:48
70	14.3 15.8	5:44 7:10	3:33:45 4:16:30
71	14.5 15.9	5:46 7:13	3:36:00 4:19:12
72	14.6 16.1	5:50 7:18	3:38:24 4:22:05
73	14.8 16.3	5:54 7:22	3:40:39 4:24:47
74	14.9 16.4	5:58 7:27	3:43:12 4:27:50
75	15.1 16.6	6:01 7:32	3:45:27 4:30:32
76	15.2 16.8	6:05 7:36	3:35:51 4:33:25
77	15.4 16.9	6:09 7:41	3:50:15 4:36:18
78	15.5 17.1	6:13 7:46	3:52:30 4:39:00
79	15.7 17.3	6:16 7:50	3:54:54 4:41:53
80	15.9 17.4	6:20 7:55	3:57:09 4:44:35

value of 1.289, and you obtain 8316.52 seconds. Alas, the differences between a time system based on 60s and a decimal system based on hundreds complicates reverse calculations, but Kelly would have run 2:18:46.

The tables also permit comparison between your times and the times of other athletes. For instance, Kelly ran 2:37:42 in Yonkers, N.Y., in 1962, placing fourth in the National AAU Championships at age 54. What is the comparative value of that performance to his time seven years later? The tables tell us his 1962 performance was worth 2:11:51, several minutes faster than the top young athletes of the world were running at that period. It was also statistically superior to his age-61-time, not to mention his all-time best performance of 2:30:00.

The following tables also include information as to how swimmers and field event performers can compute their performance values in several events. Unfortunately, there is no easy method of determining decline in ability in sports that do not lend themselves to statistical summarization, although we have included a best-guess estimate (based on statistical values for swimmers and runners) as to what that decline might be. Only after another 10 or 20 years, as more and more older athletes continue in the competitions of their youths, will we be able to judge the true accuracy of these charts.

General Slowdown

(Can be applied to most middle-distance running events such as the mile, as well as to swimming events. Most other fitness activities probably would also follow this same drop in efficiency.)

Age	Decline %	Age	Decline %
35	3.0	58	25.3
36	3.6	59	26.6
37	4.2	60	28.0
38	4.8	61	29.4
39	5.5	62	30.8
40	8.1	63	32.3
41	7.0	64	33.8
42	7.8	65	35.3
43	8.7	66	36.8
44	9.5	67	38.3
45	10.4	68	39.8
46	11.3	69	41.3
47	12.2	70	42.8
48	13.1	71	44.3
49	15.0	72	45.9
50	15.2	73	47.4
51	16.4	74	49.0
52	17.6	75	50.5
53	18.8	76	52.1
54	20.1	77	53.7
55	21.4	78	55.2
56	22.7	79	56.7
57	24.0	80	58.3

Slowdown Table for the 100 Meters

Age	Decline %	Age	Decline %
35	4.7	58	25.9
36	5.3	59	27.2
37	6.0	60	28.6
38	6.7	61	30.0
39	7.4	62	31.4
40	8.1	63	32.9
41	8.8	64	34.4
42	9.6	65	35.9
43	10.3	66	37.3
44	11.0	67	38.8
45	11.8	68	40.2
46	12.6	69	41.7
47	13.3	70	43.2
48	14.1	71	44.7
49	15.0	72	46.2
50	16.0	73	47.8
51	17.1	74	49.3
52	18.2	75	50.8
53	19.4	76	52.3
54	20.7	77	53.9
55	22.0	78	55.4
56	23.3	79	56.9
57	24.6	80	58.5

Slowdown for the Marathon

Age	Decline %	Age	Decline %
35	1.3	58	24.8
36	1.9	59	26.1
37	2.4	60	27.5
38	3.0	61	28.9
39	3.7	62	30.3
40	4.5	63	31.8
41	5.3	64	33.3
42	6.2	65	34.8
43	7.1	66	36.3
44	8.0	67	37.9
45	9.0	68	39.4
46	10.1	69	41.0
47	11.1	70	42.5
48	12.2	71	44.0
49	13.3	72	45.6
50	14.5	73	47.1
51	15.7	74	48.8
52	17.0	75	50.3
53	18.3	76	51.9
54	19.6	77	53.5
55	20.9	78	55.0
56	22.2	79	56.6
57	23.5	80	58.1

Slowdown for Throwing Events

There is a basic difference between running events and throwing (or field) events that probably should be pointed out. Times increase in the former whereas distances decrease in the latter. Ken Young also noticed that as ages increased, throwers seemed to decline much more precipitously than runners. He speculated that as we grow older we continue to use our legs in normal activities, but are less likely to use our arms. To obtain your optimum performance in an event such as the shot put, you would multiply your distance by the appropriate figure below. For example, a shot putter aged 45 would multiply his performance by 1.152.

Age	Decline %	Age	Decline %
35	5.8	58	35.0
36	6.7	59	37.1
37	7.6	60	39.1
38	8.5	61	41.1
39	9.4	62	43.2
40	10.4	63	45.3
41	11.3	64	47.4
42	12.2	65	49.5
43	13.2	66	51.6
44	14.2	67	53.7
45	15.2	68	55.8
46	16.3	69	57.9
47	17.4	70	59.9
48	18.6	71	61.9
49	19.8	72	63.8
50	21.1	73	65.6
51	22.5	74	67.3
52	24.0	75	69.0
53	25.6	76	70.6
54	27.3	77	72.1
55	29.1	78	73.6
56	31.0	79	75.1
57	33.0	80	76.5

Part Three:
FOOD AND FITNESS

9

The Battle Of the Bulge

One overweight friend of mine named John tells a story about his efforts to enlist in the Navy during World War II. When he appeared at the recruiting station, his belt all but invisible, the officer winced, eyed him clinically, then finally said, "Go home and lose 20 pounds."

Love of country motivated John to great dietary accomplishments. On his second trip to the recruiting station, the officer said, "Now go home and lose 20 *more* pounds." That accomplished, he was told to remove a still additional 20 pounds.

Before reaching this goal, however, John collapsed and was rushed to the hospital—suffering from malnutrition and weighing 237 pounds! No Purple Heart was issued.

"I live happily with no frustrations until I gain so much weight I can't get into my clothes," he told me recently. "I have three separate wardrobes. I diet until I can fit into the middle set, then relax until they're snug. Then I diet some more until I can get into the next set. Occasionally, I have gone out and bought a new suit that is too small and dieted into it, using the clothes as both incentive and reward. Ordinarily, I diet continuously, starving myself all day until I'm confident by nightfall that I have lost at least nine pounds. Then as a reward for being so good, I eat a big snack before bed."

John would seem to be among the majority of Americans. According to a survey conducted some years ago by Alfred Politz Research, Inc., for the makers of a diet food, 58% of the adult population in America was overweight. Assuming those figures are current, if every adult in the United States were at this very moment to stand naked in the bathroom with a ruler in one hand and the skin of the belly in the other (the famous "pinch" test), 130 million would be grasping more than an inch of blubber. Moreover, according to Politz, 33% of the adult population, or 79 million people, are "concerned about being overweight," one reason for the currently booming diet industry. Americans spend billions of dollars on low-calorie foods each year, and some of the most popular soft drinks today are low-calorie ones.

But the question might be raised: Should people interested in fitness lose weight?

Not if they are going to regain it. "Temporary weight loss is of no value," claims the American Medical Association. "There is ample evidence that an individual staying with a diet will lose weight. But most people eventually abandon the diet and rapidly regain their lost pounds. Obviously, they didn't learn anything. And when they return to their former weight, they may be in poorer shape, both physically and medically, than before. A person who constantly gains, loses, gains, then attempts to lose again may actually be shortening his life. We simply don't know."

There are many unanswered questions about dieting. For example, take longevity. The rewards for being slim include a longer life. Overweight is one of the 10 risk factors, as listed earlier (Chapter Three) by Dr. Herman K. Hellerstein. According to the National Heart Institute, the risk of heart attack is five times greater for a man with high cholesterol levels—10 times greater if he is overweight. Insurance statistics indicate the death rate for overweight men to be 79% higher than for men of normal weight. Medical researchers can point to a direct coorelation among obesity, diabetes and heart disease.

"Obesity isn't a disease," says a spokesman for the American Medical Association. "You don't die from obesity. You die from heart disease or your kidneys give out. You die from the *complications* of obesity."

Most nutritionists agree that the thin man will outlive the fat man. But nobody yet has effectively proved that the fat man will live longer if he attempts to become thin.

Some years ago, a British researcher named R. F. J. Withers published a study which dropped like a bomb in the laps of nutritionists. Withers studied the weight differences of both the natural and adopted children of obese parents in a south London suburb. He discovered that the natural children usually were fat like their parents. The adopted children, however, often were slim.

"This shook up a lot of us," admits the AMA spokesman. "Many of us had assumed people were fat only because they ate too much. They figured that fat parents had fat children because the kids adopted their eating patterns. Thus, obesity was caused mostly by environment. But studies by Withers and other researchers challenged this traditional view. It pinned obesity, or a tendency toward obesity, to heredity. People were fat at least in part because of their genetic makeup."

(Or they were fat, as others suggested later, because the poor nutritional habits of their mothers during pregnancy stigmatized them and established a craving for certain types of nutrition that they would carry with them into adult life.)

Thus, attempts to mold people into what may be an unnatural size and weight seemingly must meet with disaster. Statistics seem to bear this out. Studies by TOPS (a Milwaukee-based organization with initials meaning "Take Off Pounds Sensibly") show that 47% of dieters quit after one year; 70% after two years. Fewer than 2% maintain weight loss for five years. Officials at the American Medical Association suggest that only about 5% of dieters are successful. They define success not merely as taking weight off, but *keeping* it off.

"Occasionally, you see studies where they have had success ratios of 40-50%," says one physician, "but usually this reflects only six months or so of research. You check back a few years later and find that the percentage of those who have maintained their loss has shrunk considerably."

TOPS rates as the calorie-counter's equivalent of Alcoholics Anonymous, although according to founder Esther Manz, "There is nothing anonymous about being fat." Esther Manz weighed 208 pounds in 1948 when her doctor told her to reduce. Rather than suffer alone, she enlisted the aid of three 200-plus friends, and a *Milwaukee Journal* article describing their eventual success inspired others to form similar groups. The movement spread slowly at first, but there are presently 12,000 TOPS chapters functioning in all 50 states plus 27 other countries. Its 300,000 members lost a collective two million pounds last year. The 1976 champion calorie-counter was Kay Abell of Watertown, N.Y., who in 12 months descended from a corpulent 311 pounds to a svelte 150. Yale Browstein of Chicago dropped from 370 pounds to 190.

"TOPS pretends to be neither spiritual nor miraculous," claims Manz. "We're just a plain sensible organization for helping people get weight off." The success rate of this self-help and non-profit group easily exceeds that of persons dieting alone or that of the wealthy few who can indulge themselves in plushly decorated reducing parlors.

According to diet consultant Ted Berland (who has written a book, *Rating the Diets*), "Middle-aged people mostly have a weight problem because of their lack of exercise and their abundance of food. Men, particularly, revel in their sports days in high school or college, and seem to forget that 20 years have slid by and the closest they get to any active sports is their TV screen.

"They also are likely to be in business or professions or trades, where there is ample opportunity to eat, especially if they are on expense accounts. The business lunch becomes a ritual, often preceded by a calorie-rich drink. Women put their weight on with each pregnancy, especially if they do not breast-feed their babies. Furthermore, the temptations are ever-present in kitchen, and as their husbands work harder and longer to buy food, the women grow lonelier in their kitchens and nibble more.

"Many middle-aged men and women think they have a right to get fat, since their body metabolism is slowing down. What actually has slowed down is their oomph. Their body metabolism slows down negligibly once they achieve full maturity and height."

Many physicians shudder when they see a fat person walking in the door to plead for a reducing diet. "The doctors know the odds," sighs Berland, "and they dislike having to participate in another person's failure."

Most doctors probably fail to realize what a major catastrophe being fat can be to many people. For that same reason, the amount of medical research that has been directed toward the problem of curing obesity is negligible when compared with amounts spent for diseases such as cancer and polio.

Because of the admitted lack of thorough research, many dietitians find they must respond to direct questions with qualified "maybes" and "ifs."

"You get much more authoritative answers from the quacks and food faddists," says Ted Berland. "They think everything is either black or white. We know there are a lot of variables."

The problem of what even is "plump" is difficult to resolve. Insurance weight charts can serve only as a guide. They represent averages, and not all healthy people conveniently can be matched against averages. One airline that tried to make the weight of all its stewardesses conform to insurance tables found itself with a revolt on its hands. The airlines lost, and perhaps those of us who frequently travel by air can be thankful. Life probably should consist of a little pasta.

In addition to the grossly overweight, there exists also the grossly underweight. Approximately 10 million Americans need to *add* rather than subtract pounds, *if* you rely on insurance standards. My mother-in-law thinks I'm skinny and always is trying to fatten me up. The American philosophy is that plump is beautiful—as long as it is not too plump. This is one reason why the greatest percentage of those overweight often are in the middle class who consider plumpness a sign of prosperity. The poorest in the lower class may be thin from starvation. Those in the upper class may not need food to symbolize their prosperity.

The best advice to offer dieters is to be consistent. According to Ted Berland, "Better to stay overweight than to wage the seesaw battle that fat people wage—first dieting, then stuffing themselves."

This often puts undue stress on heart and arteries. Doctors also suspect that repeated attempts and failures at dieting may affect a person psychologically. Each failure to achieve what the insurance companies consider a healthy weight may lower a person's esteem of himself just one more notch.

Dietitians are uncertain as to why some people gain weight and others do not, even with apparently identical intakes of calories. Many thin people seemingly can shovel food down their mouths without gaining an ounce. A fat person, on the other hand, may be unable to eat more than half the thin person's calorie load without bulging enormously. (Of course, many fat people conveniently "forget" to include snacks and nibbling in their daily calorie counts.)

Many fat people insist that their metabolism *is* different, but this is not true; both fat and thin people expend calories in the same manner.

"It's a balance," says one physician. "You have caloric intake on one hand and caloric expenditure on the other. That part is easy. There's no ambiguity. What we don't understand is why people get out of balance."

Apparently, many fat people, whether because of heredity or not, burn fewer calories than do thin people in the normal act of day-to-day living. They find it easier to sit quietly in a chair. They don't tap their feet to music. They take life more calmly and thus do not feel compelled to take stairs two at a time. Instead, they wait for the elevator.

"What it amounts to," asks Ted Berland, "is, are you or aren't you a swinger?"

Those who are not swingers find themselves trapped in a vicious circle. Being initially less active they gain weight, which immobilizes them further, which makes it easier for them to gain more weight. A thinner person can exercise more comfortably than a fat person and therefore finds it easier to remain thin.

A similar vicious circle exists in the psychological area of overweight. Fat people find themselves discriminated against in many areas because of their weight, so they eat more as a salve for their hurt feelings.

People able to buy their clothes off the racks in department stores probably do not realize the many subtle ways in which fat people are discriminated against. One study showed a higher percentage of fat people in the freshman year of high school than in the freshman year of college, indicating (taking grades and intelligence into consideration) that college admissions officers, whether consciously or subconsciously, may be discriminating against applying students because of their weight and appearance. In one psychological study of girls in a weight-reduction camp, the girls were found to exhibit personality characteristics strikingly similar to those recognized by social anthropoligists to be typical of ethnic and racial minorities subject to discrimination.

According to the American Medical Association's Dr. Philip L. White, "We're past the era when obesity was the sign of success. In the past, I suspect many of our American Presidents were overweight. That day is gone. The present-day executive is a lean, trim, hardy, ruddy individual."

Pollster Louis Harris deduced that suburban residents worry more than any other group about their weight. According to a survey conducted by the Department of Psychiatry at the University of Pennsylvania, obesity was six times more common among women of low status than with those of high status.

"Furthermore," states the study, "upwardly mobile females were less obese (12%) than the downwardly mobile (22%)."

Again, the question might be asked: Do people reach high status because they are slim or do the same personality traits which cause them to be successful in other areas also cause them to be successful dieters? Beyond that, maybe upwardly mobile men like their wives skinny.

The majority of dieters are women: about 80%. However, at least in the area of the grossly obese, men usually prove to be better dieters than women—they achieve success more often—perhaps because the necessity to advance in their jobs provides motivation. Furthermore, the typical dieters are not persons 40 or 50 pounds overweight, but more likely individuals 5-10 pounds overweight who diet to remain within at least striking distance of what they consider to be a good figure. It is them that the billion-dollar diet industry serves.

In fact, the mid-20th century version of the better mousetrap cliche goes: Devise a better diet and the world will beat a path to your door. Dr. Atkins and Dr. Stillman have made millions from their best-selling diet books. In fact, the two most popular categories on the best-seller list year after year (if you exclude Bibles) are: (a) diet books, and (b) cook books (not necessarily in that order).

Metrecal, a liquid 225-calorie diet substitute, did business at the rate of $120 million annually in the early 1960s and spawned several hundred imitators before it lost fashion as people tired of that approach to losing weight.

Medical authorities smiled pleasantly on liquid diets, when they first appeared, but their eyebrows curl, their nostrils dilate and their jaws shudder as they contemplate the many less responsible reducing gimmicks. So many are the money-making schemes—pills that "melt weight off," candy that when taken before meals supposedly satiates the appetite, the many reducing salons (for the "rich obese")—that watchdog organizations like the Food and Drug Administration, the Postal Service, the Better Business Bureau and the American Medical Association have difficulty even thinning out the ranks of the faddists, much less controlling them. Also difficult to control are reducing schemes and diets which do not constitute fraud as much as they constitute simply bad advice.

Probably the most universally condemned fad in the past few decades was the *Drinking Man's Diet*, a book published in paperback that reportedly sold around 10 million copies. Actually the "Drinking Man's Diet" was just another in a still-continuing series of more or less similar low-carbohydrate weight-loss regimens that apparently originated with the Banting Diet in England 100 years ago and continued through the DuPont Diet of the 1940s, the Taller (or "Calories Don't Count") Diet of 1961 and Atkins' "Diet Revolutions" of the 1970s. All suggested that by lowering daily carbohydrate intake to below 60 grams, the dieter could forget about his intake of calories. In theory, some magic of body chemistry caused fat to vanish. This relieved the overweight person of the bothersome bookkeeping chores such as calorie counting, and supposedly he could eat and drink as much as his fat little heart desired. But in actual practice, if his caloric intake failed to drop, neither would his weight.

According to Ted Berland, author of *Rating the Diets*, the hottest new diet is the *Last Chance Diet*, a book by osteopath Dr.

Robert Linn and writer Sandra Lee Stuart. The book promotes the use of a liquid protein named Pro-Linn (protein plus Linn). Health food stores now sell imitations.

"Supposedly this should be taken under a doctor's care, but the item as a food is non-prescription," says Berland.

Also popular are the various fiber diets which are based on the (unproven and unscientific) premise that lots of fiber in food will speed it so fast through the intestines that they will not be able to absorb many nutrients. Fasting, a quick, sure and sometimes dangerous way to lose weight, has also become popular. Ear acupuncture remains another fad.

"It (acupuncture) works," smiles Berland, "only if the person with the staple in the ear sticks to a low-calorie diet."

The amount of advice available to the dieter is, indeed, overwhelming, both in magazines and books. "I think many of our popular magazines, particularly the women's magazines, are editorially irresponsible when it comes to printing information on diets," I was told by Dr. Frederick J. Stare of Harvard University's Department of Nutrition.

"It's too bad that editors feel such a compulsion to please their readers," adds Dr. White. "As for authors, often when they put in the three words, 'See your doctor,' they think they have absolved themselves of all responsiblity for editorial content."

If obesity is related to heredity, rather than environment, and if a fat person may injure himself either physically or mentally by repeated failures to become thin, then such attention to diets would be ill-advised. Many nutritionists believe that the present generation of fat people may already be lost, so they hope to achieve more success by concentrating their efforts on the coming generations who can learn better dietary habits both through instruction and example.

The ultimate secret of any permanent weight-reduction program is not to deprive yourself of so-called "fattening foods" (all foods are fattening) but simply not to eat as much of them. A diet should be appetizing to be successful, which would seemingly rule out most bizarre diets that appeal to the dieting public.

"A person has to lose weight without thinking of himself as a suffering individual," says a spokesman for the AMA. "He has to learn new and improved dietary habits. This is one reason why crash diets fail. People can't stay on them indefinitely. They may meet their needs for nutrients, but not their psychological needs. Two months is a minimum time for retraining dietary habits, and in most people it may take longer. If a person continues to think of himself as dieting, he has not gone over to the winning side."

10
The Miracle Diet Doctor Of the Mountains

In his job of trying to shrink pounds off people through exercise, Marcus Sorenson, Ph.D., director of the National Institute of Fitness, frequently encounters apologetic clients.

"I can't follow your program," they say. "I'm simply not athletic."

Dr. Sorenson refuses to accept this excuse. He insists, "Unless you *get* athletic and play some game, or do something physically, you will fail!"

He explains his position: "There is no way anybody with an overweight problem can stay thin without exercise. Statistics show that obese people get thin occasionally by dieting, but they always return to their previous weight unless they add that magic ingredient: exercise."

Use of that magic ingredient has resulted in miracle cures for many of those who have participated in Dr. Sorenson's weight reducing programs, either at his summer center in the mountains near Cedar City, Utah, or at his winter center in Tempe, Ariz.

One Phoenix attorney lost 52 pounds in 56 days. He is now on a racquetball program to lose 50 additional pounds. A woman from Portland, Ore., lost four dress sizes in two weeks. A man from Denver, Colo., shed 21 pounds in nine days. A lawyer from California arrived at Dr. Sorenson's camp barely able to jog 10 yards. Sixty pounds lighter, he now runs a half-mile faster than four minutes. World-class athletes travel twice the distance in that time, but, as Dr. Sorenson points out, success is relative.

Those, admittedly, are some of Dr. Sorenson's more noteworthy success stories, but he can point to a success ratio for his clients of 50%—much higher than that achieved at better publicized and more expensive diet health spas that cater to the wealthy. He often receives letters from former clients who say, "I lost another 20 pounds."

Yet, a 50% success ratio also indicates a 50% *failure* ratio, something that Dr. Sorenson sadly concedes. Those who fail rarely write. "If they don't go home and get active like I tell them," Dr. Sorenson admits, "they are going to come back to me heavier or go someplace else heavier." He says he prefers not to see his clients again: "I would rather see their overweight friends."

Most physicians warn against too rapid weight loss, for good reason. More than fat is lost on any crash diet. An individual who suddenly stops eating and loses, say, 60 pounds will shed two or three pounds almost immediately by draining excess body liquids. Thirty or 40 pounds of body fat will disappear. But the remainder of the loss will be lean body mass: muscles, bone, glands and blood.

"This is why people who starve themselves look terrible," explains Dr. Sorenson. "Their skin hangs loose. They get wrinkles. They seem pale. They become weak. They appear to be in bad health and, in fact, *are* in bad health."

Should their will-power dissolve, these starvation dieters face another problem. When they return to the banquet table and regain their lost 60 pounds, they will regain mostly fat, possibly as much as 50 pounds. Most of the lean body mass lost during their diet will not be recovered immediately. Once they look at themselves in the mirror and start pushing food away again, they risk losing still more lean body mass. This is why persons who yo-yo, allowing their weight to constantly go up and down, can severely damage their health.

But add the miracle ingredient, exercise, along with diet, and the body no longer loses lean body mass as it shrinks. On the contrary, it *adds* lean body mass. The muscles strengthen. The bones become stronger. Red blood cells begin to proliferate, stimulated by the exercising body's need for more oxygen. The result is better, rather than poorer, health.

One woman from Mesa, Ariz., lost 41 pounds during a 41-day stay at Dr. Sorenson's camp in Utah. Actually, skin-fold measurements indicated that she lost *51* pounds of body fat. Her exercise regimen built 10 pounds of muscle. Similar results occur among other of Dr. Sorenson's clients who exercise as they diet.

"Another beautiful thing about exercise," he suggests, "is that it depresses the appetite. People who exercise vigorously for an hour and a half a day, according to studies by Dr. Jean Mayer of Harvard, ingest fewer calories."

Long-distance runners have known this to be true even before Harvard researchers proved it. A runner who comes in from a hard workout and sits down at the dinner table often finds himself picking at his food rather than reaching for a second helping.

I first got to know Marc Sorenson during the summer of 1976 when I visited Runner's Mecca, a high-altitude training camp for distance runners directed by Rich Heywood, track coach at Mesa (Ariz.) high school.* Runner's Mecca was located at an altitude near 10,000 feet in the shadow of Brian Head, a mountain which during the winter provides the focus for a popular ski area. We stayed in Chalet Village, across the road from the ski slope.

There were up to a hundred of us runners, mostly high school athletes preparing for cross-country. I was a guest lecturer. We ran twice daily, five or 10 miles a workout, along the roads or through the woods. Also sharing Chalet Village with us, however, were the "Niffies" (as we called them), the term coming from the intitials of National Institute of Fitness. We used the term fondly, not derisively, since the Niffies also were engaged in physical activity, although at a lower level. They received their meals from

---

* The theory behind high-altitude training is that by living and running at altitudes above 5000 feet, you stimulate your body to produce additional oxygen-carrying red corpuscles. When you return to sea level, supposedly you have super-charged blood and can defeat runners of equal ability who are not altitude trained.

a menu carefully planned by Marc Sorenson and served at a small restaurant up the road named Ferdinand's. The fact that the restaurant was apart from their living quarters forced the Niffies to walk a half-mile uphill (breakfast, lunch or dinner) to be fed, then a half-mile down afterwards. Most walked farther.

Rich Heywood introduced me to Marc Sorenson, and I also met several of the Niffies. Many of them joined in our volleyball games—or maybe it was us joining in their volleyball games. They went for long walks in the tree-green high country of southern Utah. We were only a few miles away from Cedar Breaks National Monument, which is every bit as stunning as the Grand Canyon or Zion National Park. The scenery encouraged you to get out and enjoy it. The air may have been thin, but it was clean.

Each morning, the Niffies would appear outside Dr. Sorenson's apartment to check their weight and record their progress. He also did occasional skin-fold tests, using calipers to estimate percentage of body fat. A man who has 20% or a woman with 25% body fat is considered "obese." Most of the Niffies far exceeded those percentages—at least when they arrived in camp.

Because my wife was interested in losing several pounds during our two-week stay at Runner's Mecca, she also occasionally joined the Niffies for their ritual morning weigh-ins. She found them pleasant and friendly. In general, the runners and dieters got along well since both groups were pursuing the same basic goal: physical fitness.

One reason, other than scenery, that Dr. Sorenson selected the high-altitude location was that in the rarified atmosphere of 10,000 feet the body metabolism works harder to assure a sufficient oxygen supply for the muscles. "You use more calories in the simple act of breathing than you would at sea level," he explained. The cool air also was an attraction to vacationing dieters from Arizona and Southern California who wanted to escape the heat of the summer. But the most important factor was the isolation of the camp. Dr. Sorenson said, "I thought the only way people could succeed in getting thin was for me to remove them from their environment and bad habits, and hopefully teach them something about losing weight."

That was during the summer. In the winter, he rents a dozen units in an apartment complex in Tempe, Ariz. But while he originally expected the warm-weather winter camp would appeal mostly to people from cold cities and the cool-weather summer camp would appeal to people from hot cities, he finds his clients come from everywhere, at all times, to both camps. "The main attraction seems to be losing weight," he stated.

When I visited him in Tempe one afternoon in January 1977, he was relaxing after a vigorous morning of activities with his Niffies. Following breakfast, they played racquetball for an hour, attended an exercise class, then took a four-mile walk. After lunch, they planned to meet on the lawn and throw frisbees and kick-balls around before listening to a lecture by Dr. Sorenson on the physiology of fat. On other days, they play volleyball and engage in water sports. The next day, he planned to take them to South Mountain for a long hike in the park. On Sunday, they would take a 15-mile hike from the top of that mountain back to camp.

"The main thing I'm interested in is just to keep them moving," Dr. Sorenson explained. "I want to keep their minds off food, because they don't get much to eat." Meals for those staying at his Tempe camp were provided at a nearby restaurant called the Jolly Roger, also from menus designed by Dr. Sorenson.

"They have to make one of two choices," he continued. "They've got to be hungry all their lives or they've got to be active. If they choose to be active, they can eat a lot more and still not gain weight. This enables them to enjoy the food they love so much."

He feels that, particularly in the last century, man has allowed his amount of energy expended and the amount and quality of food consumed to get out of balance. In lectures before his groups, Dr. Sorenson frequently refers to the caveman hundreds of thousands of years ago who, if he wanted meat for a meal, had to chase an animal and club it. Sometimes animals chased him. So he obtained sufficient exercise. Otherwise, he grubbed for roots or ate fruits and berries off the trees. Man thus evolved by obtaining ample exercise and eating natural foods.

At the turn of the century, with the increased development of machines, man became more sedentary. He exercised less. At the same time, he began to eat more refined foods: white sugar, white flour, frozen fruit juices instead of actual fruit. The combination of a diet laden with refined foods and lack of physical activity caused his health to deteriorate. He became plagued by various degenerative ailments. Heart disease, virtually unheard of before the 20th century, became common because of arteries clogged with fatty deposits from rich foods. Cancer increased because of the ingestion of preservatives, not to mention the effects of air pollution and cigarette smoking. Diabetes is now on the rampage because of increased sugar consumption.

Twentieth-century man also increased in weight. In his lectures, Dr. Sorenson talks about reactive hypoglycemia, what might in layman's terms to be described as the "Coffee Break Syndrome." A person begins the day with a big breakfast which raises the level of his blood sugar. This is all right since a certain level of blood sugar is necessary to provide energy. But if the breakfast consisted of too many refined carbohydrates—such as sugar on the grapefruit, sugar in the coffee, jelly on the toast—the blood sugar level will raise too high. This triggers an insulin reaction. The pancreas shoots extra insulin into the bloodstream in order to metabolize the excessive sugar. But the sugars feeding into the bloodstream from the sugar-rich breakfast quickly ceases, and the insulin gland continues to work, overshoots the need and lowers the blood sugar level too much.

This causes the person to feel let down, so at 10 in the morning he takes a coffee break, using several teaspoons of sugar in the coffee, perhaps also eating a sweet roll or doughnut. This temporarily raises the blood sugar level again, triggering still another insulin reaction which lowers it. An expansive lunch, followed by another coffee break, followed by a large dinner, followed by an evening snack before bed, followed by a midnight snack results in excessive calorie intake. It also produces a roller-coaster effect on the blood sugar level, which eventually can fatigue the pancreas and be a contributing factor to diabetes. But a more frequent result of this Coffee Break Syndrome is obesity.

By age 50, one out of every two women in the United States is obese (meaning more than 25% body fat), and one out of every three men is obese (more than 20% body fat). Another one out of every four individuals is significantly heavier than necessary.

Dr. Sorenson states, "I've heard that at Brigham Young University, the average college co-ed gains between 28 to 32 pounds during her four years on campus." He shakes his head sadly.

Approximate Metabolic Cost of Activities

The following list of the number of calories burned in different physical activities was prepared by Robert E. Johnson, M.D., and colleagues from the department of physiology and biophysics at the University of Illinois in August 1967. It was published in a booklet prepared by the American Medical Association entitled, *Basic Bodywork . . . for fitness and health.*

Dr. Johnson's standards showed the gross energy expenditure in calories per hour by a 150-pound individual, and his standards represented a compromise between those proposed earlier by the British Medical Association (1950), Christensen (1953), and Wells, Balke and Van Fossen (1956). Where available he used actual measured values and otherwise made what he referred to as a "best guess."

Activity	Calories
Running (10 m.p.h.)	900
Scull rowing (race)	840
Cycling (13 m.p.h.)	660
Squash and handball	600
Skiing (10 m.p.h.)	600
Swimming (0.5 m.p.h.)	600
Hill climbing (100 feet/hour)	490
Water skiing	480
Tennis	420
Wood chopping or sawing	400
Ice skating (10 m.p.h.)	400
Ditch digging (hand shovel)	400
Table tennis	360
Roller skating	350
Volleyball	350
Square dancing	350
Horseback riding (trotting)	350
Badminton	350
Swimming (0.25 m.p.h.)	300
Walking (3.75 m.p.h.)	300
Rowing (2.5 m.p.h.)	300

Fencing	300
Lawn mowing (hand mower)	270
Bowling	270
Lawn mowing (power mower)	250
Golf	250
Canoeing (2.5 m.p.h.)	230
Walking (2.5 m.p.h.)	210
Bicycling (5.5 m.p.h.)	210
Domestic work	180
Standing	140
Driving an automobile	120
Sitting	100
Lying down or sleeping	80

"They come to BYU to get married and wonder why they fail."

He also points out that sudden death from heart attack and heart disease is three times greater among people who are obese. Vascular disease, the hardening of the arteries and atherosclerotic buildup, is three times more common. Hypertension, better known as high blood pressure (a major cause of strokes) is twice as common among obese people. Eighty per cent of diabetics were obese before contracting that disease. Obesity also is a major factor in increasing the frequency of arthritis, joint diseases, kidney diseases, cirrhosis of the liver, intestinal obstructions, hernias and suicides.

"When you add all these factors up," he concludes, "it means that if you are obese, you will live approximately seven years, on the average, less than if you were not."

In lecturing to his groups, he describes some of the methods by which people attempt to shed weight without dieting. One is by ingesting a tapeworm which will grow in your intestinal tract and digest excessive food. But while this removes the weight problem, you now have a tapeworm problem. Other individuals use a technique often used by jockeys and models, namely sticking a finger down their throat and regurgitating food right after it is eaten. (One client of Dr. Sorenson admits that she once did this immediately after falling off her previous diet with an eating binge, and became so disgusted at herself that she came to him so it would never happen to her again.) Some overweight people have had their jaws wired shut so they could not eat solid food. Others have an intestinal bypass, preventing what they eat from being adequately digested.

Another surgical technique is a lipectomy, in which a surgeon carves fat from various areas of the body. On some occasions where a lipectomy is performed on a person's belly, the result may be loss of the naval. The next step is a second operation in which an artificial naval is constructed for cosmetic reasons. The main problem occurs if the person on whom the lipectomy is performed continues to eat and replaces the surgically removed fat with new fat, which causes excessive stretching of the remaining skin. Unfortunately, there is no surgical procedure capable of removing an appetite.

Although he is a trim 165 pounds today, Marc Sorenson admits a history of overweight. Raised on a ranch along the Nevada-Utah line, he always was heavy as an adolescent. "I milked my own cow and never drank water," he says.

He played football in high school, tied several state records in weight lifting, and played racquetball, badminton and tennis. While weight lifting, he tried to increase his body weight—what weight lifters call, "bulking up." But when he got married and stopped weight lifting, along with some of his other physical activities, his weight continued to climb because of his poor eating habits.

"I know what it is like to be addicted to sugar and refined carbohydrates," he says. At age 21, he weighed 217 pounds.

He taught school and coached football for two years in California, then returned to Brigham Young for a doctorate in education with an emphasis in exercise physiology. Meanwhile, he began exercising more regularly to reduce his weight. On one occasion, he rode a bicycle 4000 miles from Phoenix to Fairbanks, Alaska. He read the book *Aerobics* and decided he needed some of that type of activity. He began to run.

Running was uncomfortable for him at first, and it took nearly seven weeks before he finally made a breakthrough in conditioning. "It happened almost overnight," he recalls. "It was like from day 42 to day 43. It suddenly felt like somebody was behind pushing me up the hill. From my physiological background, I knew what was happening. When I became more active, it caused more red corpuscles to start to form. On the 43rd day, they finally matured and went into operation. This enabled my blood to carry oxygen to my muscles with much less stress. Unfortunately, most people who start to jog for their health never get to that point. They feel uncomfortable and quit before their red corpuscles fully develop."

Through jogging and cycling, he lowered his weight to 185 pounds, a good weight for him at age 22 considering the muscles retained from his previous weight lifting. In the 10 years since, he has further reduced his weight to what he considers a more ideal 165—"although if I get careless it sometimes slides back up to 172 or 173."

He discovered one other side-benefit because of his training. Always very susceptible to colds, he often found that the cold lodged in his lungs for several weeks causing him to constantly spit up phlegm. After beginning to run, he noticed he still got colds, but the effects lasted shorter periods of time. Instead of several weeks, his lungs were free of congestion in several days.

In terms of time expended, he considers running the most efficient sport. But running is no better than any other physical activity in terms of calories burned. A person who runs a mile at a five-minute pace burns 100 calories. A person who jogs a mile at a 10-minute pace also burns 100 calories. And a person who walks a mile and takes a leisurely 20 minutes to do so still burns 100 calories.

Most long-distance runners who have these facts explained to them consider this unfair. They know the effort necessary to be able to run at a five-minute pace, something which perhaps 99% of the population of the United States is incapable of achieving. But Dr. Sorenson explains, "It takes so much energy to move a certain amount of weight through a certain space, regardless of the speed at which you do it."

Of course, a runner capable of five-minute pace can cover four miles (and burn 400 calories) in the time that the walker is covering one (and burning 100 calories). This is one reason why running is considered a more efficient form of exercise. You can burn calories faster by running and also obtain significant benefits for your cardiovascular system.

In order to lose one pound, a person must run (or jog, or walk) 35 miles, which scares some people away from exercise, since they reason this seems like too much effort for too little return. But stated in another manner, if you walk one mile a day, you can lose one pound in only 35 days; 10 pounds can be shed in a year—assuming you keep your caloric intake constant. Increase the distance run (or jogged, or walked) to four miles daily, and you can lose 40 pounds in one year.

"People sometimes say that exercise is not the key to weight to control, but it definitely is," claims Dr. Sorenson. He tells his patients that counting calories is not the only answer. He finds that some of them become so obsessed with food that they are counting all the time.

He adds, "If they get involved in physical activity, they may be able to forget about counting calories. There is no panacea for all our ills, but if there is one thing that comes closest, it is physical activity."

Although he has covered distances up to eight miles on the flat and has run to the summit of Brian Head and back (six miles), Marc Sorenson does not consider himself a runner. He enjoys racquetball more and considers it one of the best means of obtaining weight loss. An hour of vigorous racquetball will burn 600-700 calories. An hour of equally vigorous running may burn more calories (eight or 10 miles, or 800-1000 calories). But Dr. Sorenson believes, correctly, that the average person will not run that far:

"You'll never get a lot of people running. They will start, but they won't stay with it. But a person will play a game for an hour, so in that sense a game may prove superior in terms of weight loss than running, simply because a person will stick with it."

In terms of both enjoyment and weight loss, Dr. Sorenson finds he gets the most out of playing one-on-one basketball against an evenly-matched opponent.

Dr. Sorenson opened his weight reduction center at Brian Head in August 1974, attracting people by advertisements in newspapers throughout the Southwest and West Coast. "Lose Thirty Pounds," said his ads in large headlines. "No Will-Power Required." The finer print beneath the headlines explained the philosophy behind his program.

Thirty people appeared that first year, and his National Institute of Fitness has increased in popularity ever since, although he hardly threatens the success of more fashionable slimming spas such as La Costa, Golden Door and Maine Chance, which charge their clients as much as $1000 a week for weight reduction programs. Dr. Sorenson charges his clients $200 a week.

In the summer of 1976, 90 people enrolled in his program at Brian Head, and in the winter of 1976-77, 60 people appeared in Tempe. Frequently, there would be only a dozen or more people at a time staying at either camp. The National Institute of Fitness, despite its rather overreaching name, still remains small enough so that Dr. Sorenson is the one and only counselor. This may change since a $40,000 advertising campaign planned for the summer of 1977 should cause a significant increase in business.

His only major problem last summer was that non-smokers in the van riding to activities resented smokers lighting cigarettes. They kept rolling down the windows. The smokers resented non-smokers telling them they could not smoke. Dr. Sorenson hopes to solve this problem in future seasons by placing a "Thank You For Not Smoking" sign in his van.

He has definite views about what foods work best, and eats no sugar, including brown sugar or honey. He tries to avoid oils as much as possible. Even unsaturated vegetable oils (if hydrogenated) lately have become suspect, identified by research chemists as capable of clogging arteries with fat deposits much more than previously suspected.

"I never butter my bread anymore," Dr. Sorenson admits, "and I'm finding out I enjoy it just as much." He also enjoys cracked wheat cereal, grinding the wheat himself into a mush which he then sweetens with raisins and bananas. The menus which he prepares for his dieters include foods which, taken in greater portions, would probably benefit competitive athletes as well as ordinary people interested in their health.

Knowing that I was a long-distance runner, he conceded that I could be less careful about the type and quantity of foods I ate—as long as they had enough vitamins and minerals. Because of my excessive energy requirements in training for competitive races, any "garbage" ingested would quickly be burned and not result in overweight. But he also cautioned me that most marathon runners who sought to increase their performance by the now popular system of carbohydrate loading were probably going about it the wrong way.

Years ago, the typical pre-event training meal for athletic contests was a large steak, the assumption being that protein built muscles. In reality, anything eaten immediately before an athletic contest would not get digested fast enough to do much good and simply might cause the body to expend energy on digestion which best could be reserved for the coming competition. Or it might result in hypoglycemia, the Coffee Break Syndrome discussed earlier in this chapter. A hungry athlete frequently made a better athlete, although it has taken a long time to convince football coaches (and their players) of this fact.

Athletes in endurance events, however, lately have gotten into a form of carbohydrate loading, starting as much as a week before an event such as the 26-mile, 385-yard marathon. In this form of diet, runners eat high-protein meals for three or four days early in the week, allowing their hard training to burn all the stored carbohydrates in their system. This frequently causes them to become tired, irritable.

Then several days before competition, they reduce their training and shift their diet to one that is largely carbohydrate. In its pre-race coverage of the marathon at the 1976 Olympics, ABC television showed a typical training meal of Frank Shorter consisting of massive doses of spaghetti, fruit juices and candy bars. (Frank later denied that he ate the quantities that the television network showed.)

When a competitor shifts to such a diet, his carbohydrate-starved body soaks up these carbohydrates like a sponge, retaining as much as 12% more than normal. This allows an energy reserve, which athletes need in endurance events that last beyond two hours. (For shorter events, there is probably little need for carbohydrate loading.) Distance runners typically began having last meals of spaghetti the night before important competitions.

But as Dr. Sorenson pointed out, athletes who load up on white sugar products make a mistake because the sudden high blood sugar level will trigger an insulin reaction, causing the carbohydrates to be stored as fatty tissue and cholesterol, not so easily converted into energy. This insulin reaction also may lead to reactive hypoglycemia (explained earlier), causing the athlete's blood sugar level and energy to be lower than if he had not eaten sugar at all. Spaghetti is better than simple white sugars, but being made out of white flour it still is a refined carbohydrate. There is little fiber in it, and it enters the bloodstream too rapidly to be efficiently stored, also causing reactive hypoglycemia.

The proper pre-marathon meal, according to Dr. Sorenson would be complex carbohydrates: fruits such as blueberries, cherries and apples; whole wheat bread and crackers. Endurance athletes should shift from spaghetti to fruit salads.

(When I later mentioned Marc Sorenson's theories to woman marathon runner, Joan Ullyot, M.D., she conceded that fruit might work better than spaghetti, but it also might cause disturbing digestive problems. The best advice probably is to experiment to see what works best for you. Dr. Ullyot claims that carbohydrate loading for races of less than two hours' duration is probably unnecessary. She also warns against too frequent carbohydrate loading attempts because of the effects the protein depletion stage may have on the system if attempted more than several times yearly.)

But Marc Sorenson more frequently deals with people for whom a race such as 26 miles, 385 yards is so long as to be almost incomprehensible. He deals with people for whom a mile walk each day may be more exercise than they have received in their lives.

"I try to get these people to commit themselves never to take another cookie or eat any kind of refined carbohydrate—forever. They plead that these are the things that make life worth living and ask if they could have one cookie once a week, but although I sympathize with them, I also know that one cookie will lead to two or three or more, the same way it happens with an alcoholic."

He continues, "It's a shame that most people will go through life without knowing what it is like to be physically fit. I thought I was physically fit as a weight lifter, but I wasn't. I now appreciate physical fitness, exercise and proper dieting, because when you do all that, you can say to yourself: 'I'm very special.' Not in a conceited way, but you can tell yourself that you know how to take care of your body and be able to live life to a fuller extent than most others. I guess we all think we have something going for us in doing something the others refuse to do."

Marc Sorenson concludes, "People tell me, 'You must not enjoy life at all. You don't drink. You don't smoke. You do all this running and torture yourself.' But they just don't realize the quality of life they're missing. I'm 33, and I look at so many people who graduated from high school with me, with their cigarettes and their beer bellies. I can remember how these guys looked in high school when they were young and healthy, and I think it's a shame they don't know what to do with their lives."

Athletes, as well as those who want to lose weight and keep it off should be eating the following foods:

1. Whole grain breads and cereals made without sugar, honey or any other refined sweetner such as brown sugar.

2. Skim milk products.

3. Any fresh fruit except oily fruits such as avocados and olives.

4. All fish except shellfish or fish packed in oil.

5. Chicken, turkey (skinned).

6. All vegetables.

7. Egg whites only.

No refined grain products or products with oil added should be eaten. Meat and fish should be eaten sparingly. Meat should be entirely lean. No nuts should be eaten. No egg yolk, no organ meats. No cheeses except nonfat cheeses. No oils or cream. Nothing with sugar.

11

Food for Athletes

My first encounter with the idea that athletes needed different foods than "ordinary people" came during college. I sat at a training table with other members of our cross-country team, football team or whatever team happened to be sharing the season with us.

The ordinary people from our dormitory ate dinner at 6 p.m. We athletes trooped up the hill from the stadium below to eat at 6:20. Everybody else wore shirts and ties, except on Thursday (faculty night) when they wore shirts, ties and coats. We athletes wore T-shirts: white, issued clean daily from the cage, stencilled with "Property of Carleton College Athletic Department" or something or other. It was part of the status symbol of being a jock.

We also got extra portions. At this point, a quarter-century later, I am not so certain that extra portions were so decreed by the athletic director, Wally Hass, also my track coach, or whether it was because of the waiters in the dorm happened also to be athletes, working their way through college.

The fact that athletes need more food because of greater energy, therefore caloric, expenditure seems logical even today, but there was a certain amount of mysticism surrounding the training table routine—then and now. Particularly, this was true prior to competition. During the fall, our cross-country team ran at half-time of the football games, so on those Saturdays we trooped into the dining hall, precisely at 10 a.m., four hours before our competition, to eat our last meal.

And it was always the same meal: lean beef, peas, mashed potatoes, toast with honey and tea instead of milk. I disliked tea, but as an athlete going into battle I drank the beverage, as did everyone else. Pre-competition meals were like a sacred rite, a cleansing ritual by which the athlete readied himself for his ordeal.

Nobody deviated from this routine. It was not that we felt this last meal improved our performance, but we knew the competitors from that other team, somewhere nearby and at that identical hour, were sitting down to a similar meal. Should we miss any part of the ritual, they would get an edge on us which would allow them victory.

In my senior year before the conference track and field championships in a strange town—Monmouth, Ill., as a matter of fact—we went out to breakfast, and while all of us ate our toast with honey, my roommate, Chuck Nelson, ordered pancakes. This was an outrageous act of defiance, like Martin Luther nailing his theses on the doors of the church. We edged our chairs away from Chuck, certain that any moment lightning might strike. We did not want to get singed.

That afternoon at the track meet, Chuck ran his fastest time in the mile, placing third. We congratulated him and wondered if he had stumbled across some dietary secret. It looked as though we would all be shifting to pancakes for our training meals next year. But later in the meet, tired, he tried doubling back in the 880 and failed to place. We nodded knowingly at each other. Heresy had not gone unpunished. The lightning bolt had struck. "If he only hadn't eaten those pancakes," we agreed.

Myths die slowly, and I am told that the rituals with meat and honey persist at many training tables across the land, but a wave of nutritional change has begun to sweep the halls of athletica. Long-distance runners (as well as cross-country skiers) have pioneered new approaches to pre-competition meals, particularly in the area of carbohydrate-loading (as explained in the previous chapter). Because of their high carbohydrate content, pancakes are now considered a good prelude to an endurance event. Sponsors of marathon races often host spaghetti dinners the night before. Gatorade has replaced tea on training tables.

Recently, I spoke with Hank Stram, coach of the New Orleans Saints, about what his teams ate before a football game. Before becoming a football coach, Hank played halfback at Purdue University and remembers well the pre-game jitters and the ritual feedings. Attending a Big Ten university whose teams attracted spectators in the tens of thousands, however, he often ate steak rather than lean beef. But he admitted football players ate differently today.

"There has been a dramatic change from the old steak, honey and tea routine," said Stram. "Players today eat a variety of things: ice cream, pancakes, even vegetarian diets. It's amazing what people think helps them individually."

I tried to pin Stram down as to what he now considered the ideal training meal. As though afraid to give away some secret that would cause his team a future defeat, he dodged the question.

"It helps to have a lot of ability," Hank said. "If you're bigger, stronger and tougher than the others, you don't have to worry about diet."

Later, I spoke with David L. Costill, director of the Human Performance Laboratory at Ball State University, about what athletes should eat. He, too, seemed hard to pin down.

"It's very difficult to say exactly what will work for every athlete in every sport," said Costill. "We've tried to design studies, but they are a nightmare. You come up with nothing in the end. Diets for athletes are all a big hoax. Everybody has about as much information as everybody else. That's why you get all these claims about sports nutrition, because anybody can say anything they want and nobody can dispute it."

Jack Bell of the American Medical Association's Committee on Sports disputes the benefit of a single training table for campus jocks. "Sports diets for athletes is partly status symbol," he says. "The old training table with a certain quantity of food was something the athletes got because they were athletes."

Nevertheless, it is worth considering what foods athletes eat, because presumably the same type of nutritional advice that benefitted an Olympic competitor might similarly benefit a fitness jogger. Let us consider, first, some of the myths about sports nutrition.

Myth Number One: Athletes need extra protein. This relates back to the presence of steak, or beef, on the old training table. Presumably meat gives you strength. In prehistoric days, a hungry caveman would go out and bop a sabre-toothed tiger on the head for his meal. If an athlete wants to be tough like a caveman, therefore, he also needs a tiger in his tank. A thick steak is even more American than Mom's apple pie.

In actuality, athletes need relatively little extra protein. An athlete need not make special efforts to increase his protein intake. According to the National Dairy Council, "When the caloric intake of an athlete is increased, his protein intake is proportionately increased and may be more than he actually needs. Inasmuch as protein is an expensive, and inefficient, source of energy, the athlete like the normal American relies on fats and carbohydrates for fuel for his working muscles."

A sub-myth is that excessive protein consumption helps increase muscular size and strength, one reason why many weight lifters take protein supplements. But since more than 70% of a muscle consists of water, little protein is needed to produce one pound of muscle—particularly since muscle growth occurs gradually.

According to Ellington Darden, executive director of the Athletic Center in Atlanta, "The normal varied diet supplies more than enough protein."

And steak in particular is a poor pre-event food, because of its high fat content. Fat is difficult to digest.

"Steaks are more appropriate after a game than before," suggests one dietitian.

And Fred Kahms, coach of the Purdue University swimming team, says, "A lot of people no longer believe that steaks and high-protein diets are effective before athletic activity. It takes more oxygen to metabolize a gram of protein than a gram of carbohydrate."

He adds, "The real emphasis today is to get away from fad diets. In growing kids, there may be some need for protein, but for persons 40 and over, there is real concern about high protein intake. It raises the fat level, the cholesterol level, the blood lipid level."

An athlete in training will burn up most of the foods—protein, fats or carbohydrates—that he ingests at the training table. The danger occurs if and when he retires from physical activity, yet still maintains his former eating habits.

Myth Number Two: Athletes need quick-energy foods immediately before competition. Many weight men I know go to the throwing circle carrying a bag containing a jar of honey. A quick gulp of honey and they are ready to put the shot. It is almost as though they need this quick injection of energy to allow them to perform, like the drag racer who uses highly explosive nitromethane fuel, instead of ordinary gasoline, to power his engine.

Nitromethane works for drag racers, but honey does very little physically for shot putters. It may do something for them *psychologically,* particularly if their opponent realizes he has no honey in his bag of tricks. The energy apparent in any high-sugar food simply will not get into the blood stream rapidly enough to do much good, and when it does—as we saw in the last chapter—it may trigger a hypoglycemic reaction, causing the athlete to be weaker, not stronger.

According to Ellington Darden, "There are no quick-energy foods. The energy athletes expend in competition comes from food consumed anywhere from several days to two weeks before their event. At best, eating honey before competition might provide a psychological lift if athletes think it will make them stronger or faster. At worst, eating honey might cause an upset stomach or contribute to an athlete's dehydration. This is because excess amounts of honey and other sweets tend to draw fluids from other parts of the body into the gastrointestinal tract to dilute the sugar concentration."

Thus, the athlete is much better off obtaining his boost from energy pre-stored in his body. As to when that energy should be stored, it can vary greatly from individual to individual.

David L. Costill suggests, "If you're an endurance performer, you ought to have some reasonable food intake six to eight hours before you compete, just to make sure your liver is well stocked with glycogen. If you are an explosive performer, like a shot putter or a sprinter, I don't think it makes much difference. You could have a good meal two hours before competing, because your event doesn't involve your respiration or circulation."

As the father of one son who is a tennis player, I am astounded to see what players in that sport often consume before competition, sometimes between one match and another. But tennis is an entirely different sport than mine of long-distance running. I am made uncomfortable by their dietary habits, but I don't feel entirely qualified to lecture them. What it finally boils down to is that each athlete in each individual sport should, by trial and error, determine what it the best dietary regimen for himself.

Myth Number Three: Vitamins improve performance. While lecturing at a running clinic recently, I shared the podium with a runner-physician who shall remain nameless. He used a chart to show the small difference (about one second) between a gold medal and a no-medal performance in the track distance events at the 1976 Olympics. Then he offered suggestions as to how performance might be improved. One of his suggestions was that a runner should supplement his diet with vitamins.

The runner-physician was not a megavitamin freak, but he did prescribe vitamin dosages higher than what I would have considered necessary, and higher than Joan Ullyot, M.D., (who spoke before him) considered necessary. In fact, Joan and the runner-physician differed in nearly a half-dozen areas, one of them being carbohydrate loading. The runner-physician loaded frequently and for relatively short races, something Dr. Ullyot considers to be unwise. I choose to believe Dr. Ullyot when it comes to vitamins, but the fear nags at me that the runner-physician might be onto some secret which, if practiced, might make me faster.

It is that reason, more than any other, which causes athletes to pop vitamins. Recently, Olympic marathon champion Frank Shorter stayed at my house the night before a race in my home town of Michigan City, Ind. I came upstairs to find Frank standing in the bathroom gulping a vitamin pill and taking bee pollen, or at least I think it was something like bee pollen.* I asked

---

* Before I get 200 letters asking the question, I do not know what vitamin Frank Shorter was taking, and I do not care.

Frank if he thought vitamins did him any good.

"I'm not sure," he admitted. "But I hate to think that if I don't take them, someone else might get an edge on me."

That is probably what turns most vitamin-taking athletes into label-peekers. They don't want their opponents doing something that they're not doing. Frank worries about what the East Germans are taking, while they worry about what he is taking.

A year or so ago, I asked Dave Costill if I should be taking vitamins to improve my performances. He indicated that I probably got enough vitamins from my normal, balanced diet, but suggested that if I wanted to be safe, a single multivitamin tablet a day might suffice.

So I began to take the same multivitamin my three children took each morning, one prescribed by their pediatrician. The fact that their vitamins were shaped like zoo animals did not deter me. Maybe it related back to my respect for sabre-toothed tigers. But after several months of sporadic dosing, I suddenly realized I no longer reached for the vitamin jar each morning. I lacked sufficient motivation. I was not a true believer. I still was not convinced vitamins were the hot trick.

My theory is that you become a good athlete by training twice as hard as your competition, rather than by taking secret potions. I don't think Frank Shorter won a gold medal on bee pollen. More important was his training regimen of 110-140 miles a week.

Most physiologists side with me. According to the National Dairy Council, "Most investigators do not advocate vitamin supplementation for athletes for several reasons. It is a fact that excess water-soluble vitamins cannot be stored in the body and, thus, are rapidly excreted in the urine once tissue levels are saturated. Recent studies have also revealed that vitamin C supplementation had negligible effect when compared to that of a placebo on endurance performance and rate, severity and duration of athletic injury.

"In addition, vitamin C supplementation may increase biomechanical reactions in the body that destroy vitamin B-12. The fat-soluble vitamins are retained and stored in the body, and daily supplementation of large quantities of vitamin A has been known in some instances to be very toxic and even fatal. Thus, although it may be deemed advisable to increase vitamin intake for the athlete in training, this need may be met simply when the total caloric content of a nutritionally-balanced diet is increased."

I hope readers of this book don't focus on the first half of that summarizing sentence about increasing vitamin intake, without also noticing the qualification concerning the nutritionally balanced diet providing ample vitamins.

Myth Number Four: Athletes need different foods. The athlete who seeks different foods as a secret route to success has become more prevalent today. Faddisms are frequent in dieting, and athletes are susceptible to fads as much as anyone else, perhaps more than anyone else.

Some messiahs preach vegetarian diets as one panacea to peak performance and one study by Joan Ullyot, M.D., quoted recently in *Sports Illustrated*, cited evidence that among 1000 healthy persons tested, the healthiest were vegetarians who ran, the next healthiest were non-running vegetarians, followed by runners who ate an ordinary diet, then non-runners on an ordinary diet. I'm not sure Joan believes the results of her own study, since I had lunch with her one afternoon in Gainsville and she ate meat.

If a person feels that a vegetarian regimen benefits his health and/or performance, he should not be discouraged from abandoning meat. But although it is quite possible to obtain the necessary balance of proteins, fats and carbohydrates from a vegetarian diet, more attention to your planning is required compared to if you eat what we call the normal, well-rounded diet.

There is some truth, however, to the suggestion that athletes can use *different* foods, and this relates to myth number one related to overuse of protein. Athletes in training need a higher caloric intake because of their increased energy expenditure. They can more efficiently obtain this energy from carbohydrates rather than proteins and fats. Ellington Darden suggests that 50-60% of athletes' diets should consist of carbohydrate foods, which are the most efficient and desirable sources of energy.

Endurance athletes that I know (and this includes fitness joggers as well) often comment that they seem to be eating less meat than before they became involved with athletic training. However, I think it is probably not that they are eating less meat, but that they are adding other foods in addition to meat to their diet. The meat remains the same; the percentage changes.

Myth Number Five: If a champion eats certain foods, you should eat them, too. Not any more than you should wear Jaymar-Ruby slacks because of an ad in *Esquire* that says Jack Nicklaus wears them. If you like that style of slacks, fine, but it won't improve your golf game.

The afternoon before Frank Shorter raced in Michigan City, I took him to a press conference at the First-Merchants National Bank, sponsor of our race. One of the reporters asked Frank what he planned to eat the next morning. "Probably coffee and some breakfast rolls," he responded. I saw ballpoint pens scribbling furiously in notebooks. Soon, the entire world would know Frank Shorter's secret training meal.

On the way out of the bank, I commented to Frank, "I'll have to stop off at the grocery store. We don't have any breakfast rolls in the house."

Frank made a wave of his hand to dismiss the idea: "I just said that because it was the first thing that popped into my mind."

Frank Shorter may have been victim of the most flagrant example of nutritional misinformation ever offered on American TV. Before the telecast of the Olympic Marathon by ABC from Montreal in 1976, commentator Erich Segal described for viewers Frank Shorter's pre-race meal. Segal sat at a table heaped with pancakes, orange juice, candy bars and I forget what else, supposedly representing what Shorter ate before his run that day. Judging from the size of the portions, the defensive front four of the Oakland Raiders would have difficulty downing that breakfast.

Frank explained where Erich erred: "He asked me if I planned to have pancakes for breakfast, and I replied, 'I might.' Then he asked about french toast, and I said, 'I could have that, too.' The same with orange juice, and candy bars, and rolls. But what had been *or... or... or...* in the interview got translated to *and... and... and...* before the cameras."

Frank Shorter bears no malice toward Erich Segal for the bastardization of his nutritional views: "Erich is a classical scholar. He simply likes to romanticize."

To end the story, after the race in Michigan City, and after Frank left to return to his home in Boulder, Colo. I happened to glance in the kitchen sink and discovered what he ate for his pre-race breakfast. It was toast and honey.

Jack Bell of the American Medical Association summarizes his views on foods for athletes: "Most knowledgeable people feel that a normal diet, without any vitamin supplements, works for athletes as well as non-athletes, and there is nothing special they should eat to give them extra strength or energy."

Nevertheless, athletes continue to look toward nutrition as a possible source of improved performance. Ellington Darden suggests two reasons why the athletic world remains preoccupied with myths about food:

• Enormous pressure is put on coaches and athletes to win at all costs. Athletes tend, therefore, to dream that somewhere there's a food, exercise or magic formula that will make them into overnight champions.

• Also, athletes have a tremendous desire to believe in almost anything that might improve their performances. Studies show, however, that once athletes reach a high level of skill, psychological rather than physiological factors frequently determine the limits of their performance.

Darden summarized: "Thus, if athletes truly believe that a certain food or activity will improve their performance, this food or activity will probably help them even though, physiologically, it might be of no value." This is known as the placebo effect, a placebo being a medicine given to humor the patient.

During my own athletic career, I have been among the seekers of the magic ingredient that would convert me from a plodder in the pack to one who stands on the top step hearing anthems played in his honor. I was a good performer at track distances from one mile to 10,000 meters, who converted to longer distances, including the marathon, figuring that my speed might make up for any lack of endurance.

Alas, although I could run in the lead to the 20-mile point, I often had trouble going the last six miles and 385 yards of the classic marathon distance. My first three marathon attempts were twice at Boston and once at Culver City, and in each race I was in the lead, or with the leaders, past the halfway point but failed to finish. My problem was, to use an often-quoted expression, I kept running out of gas. This is a common phenomenon among fast track runners who convert to the marathon. Women, and fitness joggers, approach the event less aggressively and experience fewer problems.

I reasoned that if I could obtain some sort of special boost of energy at the 20-mile mark, I could keep going at the same pace and become a world champion. So I tried various routines. Before one 8 a.m. race, I rose in the middle of the night and ate my pre-race meal at 4 a.m., believing that to be precisely the time I could eat and allow my food to digest to provide me with lasting energy.

Then I tried Sustagen, a liquid food supplement which I could take two, and even *one*, hour before the gun sounded. I went belching to the starting line, but still failed to improve my performance.

Next, I tried glucose tablets, purchased at an apothecary shop in London while en route home from the Kosice Marathon in Czechoslovakia. One of my competitors told me about the tablets, and I figured this was why European marathoners of that era were more successful than their American counterparts. I taped tablets to the rear of my shorts during races, taking one at prescribed intervals along the route. The magic still eluded me.

Then along came Gatorade, and I drank mid-race from plastic bottles with plastic straws (so none of the precious liquid would be spilled). My wife preceded me on route, handing me my bottle every two miles along the race. It still was difficult to detect any improvement.

Finally, I discovered the secret to running faster marathons: I worked harder in practice. That is the only magic I know that works, and it works in any sport.

But the nagging question remains: agreed, there are no secret foods for fitness, but what should be in that so-called "normal, well-balanced diet" that all the experts suggest we take?

In an attempt to answer their question, I visited a dietitian, Joanne Milkereit, who works in the Hyde Park Co-op near the University of Chicago. The Co-op supposedly is the largest, single, pure supermarket in Illinois, if not in the United States. The Hyde Park Co-op sells $13 million worth of groceries a year and contains 10,000 member families. As far as Mrs. Milkereit knows, it also is the only supermarket in the country that has a full-time dietitian on its staff.

She explains her role: "I think it is very important to have dietitians in the community, as well as in hospitals, working with well people to keep them healthy. I try to be near people when they are selecting foods."

Among her duties are writing a weekly column for the community newspaper, the *Hyde Park Herald*. She occasionally offers recipes in her column, but only rarely are they recipes for desserts, unless the latter consists mainly of fruits. She develops her recipes in the test kitchen on the selling floor of the store. She frequently holds nutritional classes there for young mothers or students who may be cooking for the first time.

"I try to encourage good food choices," she explains. "One of the things I do when I'm testing a recipe is ask: Can this be made with less sugar? Less fat? Can I use vegetable oil instead of butter? Can white flour be replaced by whole wheat flour or wheat germ? I try to modify other recipes to meet the nutritional needs of the American people."

She also has radicalized the store manager when it comes to his food choices as well as the type of foods he advertises as specials. Each week ads for the Hyde Park Co-op list eight items offering special nutritional values, and they are so tagged in the store. She tests products for the manager not only for taste, but also for ingredients, steering him away from foods with too many preservatives. In the cereal aisle, she mounts a list describing the amount of sugar in each cereal.

"That does two things," Mrs. Milkereit explains. "First, it gives customers more information about the product. Second, it gives them a reason not to buy certain cereals that are high in sugar, but poor in nutrition. I've been over there when mothers will point to the tags and tell their kids they are not going to buy that because it contains too much sugar. I'm the impartial third person that they can use as an excuse to not buy something that has been over-advertised on TV."

She also separated health foods from diet foods, which previously had been lumped together in the same section of the store. She contacted physicians and other dietitians for information on the best foods for people on special diets, then promoted those foods, making special shopping lists. Sales for special diet foods increased 400% in six months.

"That doesn't mean a whole lot to me," admits Mrs. Milkereit, "but it does mean something to our manager. And it would mean something to other grocers. Maybe my next campaign will be to go out and sell a nutrition service to other owners of supermarket chains and tell them it's worthwhile to hire somebody who knows about nutrition to offer advice on foods. This would permit them to offer something that the supermarket across the street does not offer."

One other change affected in the Hyde Park Co-op was reduction of mid-aisle displays of many non-nutritional items, such as soft drinks. Irked at having to walk past a carousel stocked with candy bars on her way into her office, she also got the manager to stock it with bags of peanuts in the shell.

"I guess we have about 400% more nuts now than we did when I first started working here," she says.

For one of her weekly columns, she interviewed coaches and athletic trainers at the high school, college and professional level. "One thing that surprised me," she commented, "was the difference in attitudes between the professional trainer and the coaches on both the high school and college level. The trainer seemed to be aware of good nutrition, but not the high school and college coaches. The one myth that still seemed to be prevalent among these people was the steak dinner, and there was this business about honey."

She felt younger athletes were receiving insufficient guidance on nutrition at a period in their lives when they should be properly educated and motivated to eat the proper foods. As a result, they grow up to become older athletes with poor eating habits.

In a survey of the eating habits of professional athletes several years ago, I spoke with Bill Bates, trainer for the Milwaukee Bucks. He felt that professional basketball players had the worst nutritional habits, often because they play four or five times a week in as many different cities.

"It's sometimes a matter of expedience," he told me. "They would either lose sleep or go hungry, and often it was the latter. The National Basketball Association diet leaves a lot to be desired, especially with teams like ours who practice every day.

It's not impossible to have good dietary habits, but you have to work at it."

He described one incident when he previously was trainer with the Philadelphia 76ers. Forward Chet Walker complained about feeling tired, so coach Dolph Schayes asked Bates to find out why.

Bates explains, "Chet seemed to be sleeping enough, but we were in Cincinnati, and I saw Chet in the hotel at noon getting a cheeseburger, french fries and a milk shake. Then, before we left for the game, I spotted him in the coffee shop eating a cheeseburger, french fries and a milk shake. After the game, I didn't see him, but next day around noon there he was with a cheeseburger, french fries and a milk shake.

"I told him, "I've seen you eating three times in the last 24 hours, and you haven't had a leafy green vegetable, haven't looked at anything like broccoli or spinach. Where do you expect to get your energy?' I suggested he start varying his diet and also buying some fruit to carry in his gym bag."

What Bill Bates was suggesting, of course, was the normal, well-balanced diet everybody talks about, but too few people understand, except when it is explained to them. I tried to get Joanne Milkereit to explain her version of the normal, well-balanced diet, and she too admitted that she could not offer a definite answer.

"Usually when I talk to people about what they should eat," she explains, "I start out by asking, what do you *like* to eat? And if they say they have to have a steak every night, and assuming that causes them no economic problems, I try to talk about other foods, like baked chicken and broiled scallops, and I talk about baked beans or something like that. If they say they like fried chicken, I might recommend oven-baked chicken just to get away from eating all that fat. And if they like steak, I might suggest their having London broil once in a while, which would be flank steak, to get away from T-bone, which would have more fat. I try and take the kinds of food and either modify the cut of meat, or modify the preparation to make suggestions as to what they might eat."

She cites the recent McGovern Report, which stated four problems with American eating habits:

1. — We eat too much fat.
2. — We eat too much sugar.
3. — We should increase our intake of complex carbohydrates.
4. — We should decrease the amount of salt we use.

She encourages people to use whole-grain bread but does not totally condemn white bread, particularly for those of lesser economic means.

"White bread is cheap," she admits, "and it is enriched with three of the B vitamins and iron." She refuses to condemn an occasional meal at McDonald's, as long as it is, indeed, occasional. "You can order orange juice there instead of a soft drink," she explains, but admits that someone who ate regularly at such quick-food restaurants, where high calories often combine with low nutritional value, might have problems. She suggests having an apple for a snack in the middle of the afternoon, or, "better yet, an orange."

As for her own athletic interests, although she has a sister (Barbara Pike of Mountain View, Calif.) who runs daily, sometimes 15 miles on the weekend, Joann Milkereit tried jogging once but after two weeks abandoned it because her joints became stiff and her skin got blotchy.* So now she does yoga to improve her muscle tone and to avoid back problems she previously felt because of inactivity. She also bicycles to work, or walks if the weather is bad.

"Exercise and diet go hand and glove," Joanne Milkereit advises. "It doesn't have to be jogging, but you need to find some exercise that fits in with your life style, even if it's riding bicycles or doing yoga, climbing stairs instead of taking elevators, walking to work instead of taking the car, or parking away and walking the last mile. That helps the weight problem, and I think that psychologically people feel better. I know that I do."

She continues to claim, however, that athletes (whether fitness or competitive) do not need special foods. They simply need the same food that produces good health in all human beings. And in closing, she summarizes what might be the most important point

---

* A common complaint heard from women who begin to jog. Had she persevered past two weeks, the blotchy skin condition and accompanying itchiness probably would have disappeared.

about food for athletes, whether Olympic stars or fitness joggers.

According to Joanne Milkereit, "One thing I tell everybody is to eat a wide variety of lightly processed foods. If you only remember that about nutrition, you cannot go too wrong."

In discussing nutrition with Marc Sorenson in the previous chapter, I asked him what was his idea of a normal, well-balanced diet. He provided me with the menu from a typical week at the National Institute of Fitness, including several choices for the dinner meal. The italicized foods, at dinner, are those he *hopes* his clients choose after hearing him lecture.

BREAKFASTS

Monday: eight ounces hot whole wheat cereal, four ounces skim milk, one ounce raisins.

Tuesday: eight ounces cracked rice cereal, four ounces skim milk, one ounce raisins or other fruit.

Wednesday: natural granola (with apple and raisins), four ounces skim milk.

Thursday: eight ounces hot cracked wheat cereal, four ounces skim milk, small piece of fruit.

Friday: toast, one cup sliced strawberries (or other naturally sweet berry).

Saturday: eight ounces whole oat cereal (rolled oats), four ounces skim milk, banana (or other fruit).

Sunday: whole grain fruit pancakes with blueberries or strawberries.

LUNCHES

Lunch is a sack meal that his guests assemble when leaving breakfast. He offers enough different items so they can vary it each day, including:

1. Two ounce piece of meat: turkey, roast beef, chicken, or cheese in combination with meat to make two ounces. (Cheese should be cheddar, not American.)

2. Four pieces of raw vegetables: carrot sticks, celery sticks, cucumber rounds, cherry tomatoes, green peppers, radishes, green onions, cauliflower or zucchini.

3. Small piece of fruit: apple, banana, grapes, orange, peach, plum, tangerine, nectarine, slice of cantalope, honeydew or water-

melon. (If the fruit is large, cut it in half.)

DINNERS

Monday: *Tostada* or hamburger patty, salad and vegetable.

Tuesday: beef stew or *stuffed tomato.*

Wednesday: *Chef's salad* or grilled cheese sandwich, salad and vegetable.

Thursday: Stuffed zucchini or *turkey, salad and vegetable.*

Friday: *Fish, salad and vegetable* or *fruit plate.*

Saturday: *Steak, salad and vegetable or one deviled egg and cottage cheese.*

Sunday: Chicken, salad and vegetable or *tuna on lettuce.*

Dr. Sorenson adds that if his guests would like to substitute a piece of fruit rather than eat either of the meal choices on any given night they should let him know.

The size of servings of such foods for an athlete in training would probably be higher than for someone attempting to lose weight, but the type of food would remain the same.

Part Four:
TRAINING FOR A LIFETIME

12

Renaissance Sportsman

While researching this book, I discovered why I never became a champion swimmer. This flash of insight occurred during a period when I was sampling a number of physical activities—racquetball, swimming, handball, skiing—trying to turn myself, at least temporarily, into an athletic Renaissance Man, a jock of all sports. This, I thought, would enable me to make some value judgments. I abandoned my usual routine of running from 4-12 miles a day and at least temporarily branched off into some of these other physical activities.

One sport I sampled was swimming. In the back of my mind, I was considering the possibility of competing in a Masters swim meet scheduled for Wauwatosa, Wisc., in mid-February. Bob Collier, the swim coach at Valparaiso University, told me about it. I wrote away for an entry blank, sending a stamped, self-addressed envelope, and called my local YMCA to find out about practice facilities.

I do not belong to my local Y mainly because for the physical activities I normally engage in—running, and occasionally cycling or tennis—I can more easily dress and shower at home, which is also where I work. If I had an office job in some big city near a YMCA, I probably would join it or some equivalent athletic club. I talked with the Y's executive director. No, the Y did not offer month-long memberships (which would have gotten me through that one swim meet). But, yes, I could come in on a one-day guest visit to sample the facilities. The cost of year's adult membership was $55—or $95 if I chose to join the special men's club (extra-plush dressing facilities, permanent lockers), which most men did. Family memberships at the Michigan City YMCA were quite reasonable: $100 and $140 annually, the latter again allowing entry to the men's club. Most smokers probably burn up more than that a year in cigarettes.

I drove to the YMCA the same day, in time for the noon swim, a 1 1/2-hour period mid-day reserved for fitness swimming as opposed to lessons or kids' splashing. A half-dozen or so other men already occupied the pool, so I showered, lowered myself into the water and chose a lane.

I am not a picture-book swimmer. I had been swimming recreationally for most of my life before Sherman Atkinson, a neighbor who once swam competitively for the University of Cincinnati, told me I should not bend my knees when I kick. So now I kick with straight legs—or try to. Maintaining concentration in the water is sometimes difficult for me.

But from time to time, I have enjoyed swimming. On several occasions in high school, I tried out for the swim team. As a kid, I liked going for long-distance swims along the Chicago lake front: swimming from one beach to another a half-mile away, visiting with friends, then swimming back. In 1969, when a torn cartilage in my knee made running impossible, I switched to the water for therapeutic reasons and worked my way up to three-quarters of a mile, swimming parallel to the shore. Then I would stop at the farthest point and walk home through knee-deep water.

At the end of that summer, knee healed, I abandoned the water and returned to running the roads, but grudgingly, and partly because of approaching cold weather. Even today, after a long run on a hot day, there is nothing more pleasurable than descending to the lake in front of my house and finishing my running workout with a few swimming strokes.

In the YMCA, I did six lengths of the 25-yard pool, pausing for a few seconds between every other length before pushing off again. Mounted on the wall beside the pool was a large clock, but I paid it no attention. After six laps, I rested, then did two more lengths. Another brief rest, and I added two more. My total swim was 250 yards, good for about two points on Ken Cooper's Aerobics chart.

I rose from the pool invigorated, thinking I must swim more regularly. I carefully had limited the length of my first swimming workout, not wishing to overdo it. (Even so, I would have stiff shoulder muscles the next day.) But the challenge of practicing another sport tempted me.

Would I be able to translate my cardiovascular efficiency as a runner into success as a swimmer? Could I bridge the gap between Masters track and Masters swimming, and be a champion in both? How many laps eventually could I endure? What speeds could I attain? I remembered an unusual event, called the "biathlon," held in Columbus, Ind., each summer where competitors ran three miles then swam a half-mile. Similar run/swims take place in other parts of the country as well. Competing in one might make an interesting goal. As I showered and dressed, I vowed to return to the swimming pool regularly. Had someone shoved a YMCA application blank under my nose at that moment, I gladly would have signed. My Type A personality was straining at the bit.

Unfortunately, the next day I remembered the reason why my frequent attempts at joining my high school swim team always ended in failure: I came down with a cold.

That had been my youthful achilles heel: usually after about a week's activity in the pool, I caught a cold serious enough to keep me out of the water. By the time I recovered, my interest had waned. Even today, I find I must limit my post-run swims during the summer, because too much underwater activity bothers my sinuses. For that reason, I usually swim sidestroke, or breaststroke, to keep my nose above water.

I could see, however, the difficulty of motivating otherwise sedentary people into accepting a life of physical activity. Their own inertia first must be overcome. To exercise in any manner, you must put out a special effort. Probably a greater barrier between me and a swimming career is that, at least during the winter months, if I want to swim I must climb in a car, drive 15 minutes to the YMCA, work out, then drive 15 minutes home. Running is simpler, because my running trails start at my back door. The best physical activity is not only one you enjoy, but one that is convenient. Swimming will continue, for me, to be an enjoyable part-time activity. But I never did make that Masters swim meet in Wauwatosa.

In the meantime, I became attracted to cross-country skiing. Interest in that sport has grown considerably in our area recently. The number of my friends who mention trying the sport seems to be increasing. There are few long or large hills in northwest Indiana. But many pleasant wooded areas, including the Dunes National Lake Shore, beckon the cross-country skier as well as runner. Usually, there is sufficient snow to permit skiing between December and February.

One recent winter day, Dick Gosswiller, a fellow freelance writer who lives in nearby Michiana Shores, Mich., called to announce that he and his wife, Marianne, planned to go cross-country skiing. Would I and my wife Rose like to join them? My immediate response was yes. I can't resist any kind of challenge. We reserved skis and boots at a local ski shop several weeks in advance. The cost would be $7.25 rental for each of us for the day (although I learned later we could have rented them at the park where we planned to ski for only $3 for four hours).

On a Sunday afternoon in February, we drove to Bendix Woods near South Bend with Lou Donkle, another neighbor, middle-aged, who had been cross-country skiing the previous day, just having purchased new equipment. Lou bubbled with enthusiasm.

"It was great getting out in the fresh air," he said. "The scenery was beautiful. I enjoyed the sport enormously. I came home totally invigorated. It made me feel like I could live to be a hundred!"

(It made *me* feel like I was experiencing *deja vu*. Lou sounded like any one of at least 300 newborn runners I know.)

We arrived at Bendix Woods, at one time the test track for Studebaker Automotive Company. The snow was deep, clean.

Various two-track paths led off into the woods. Lou began offering some basic instruction to the others, but I was impatient. I wanted to be off gliding between the evergreen trees, churning up the hills with powerful strokes of my arms, swooping down the slopes: slide, glide, slide, glide. I visualized myself as Bill Koch, winning a silver medal in the Olympics. But why settle for silver? Maybe I could bridge the gap between cross-country running and cross country skiing.

Later, my companions remarked at how quickly I seemed to pick up the sport that day, but many of the body movements in cross-country skiing resemble those of cross-country running—or hurdling, which I do when running the 3000-meter steeplechase. When your left leg goes forward, your left arm goes back. The same with right leg and arm. It is step, push, step, push, and you're off through the woods. Most runners could pick up the fundamentals of cross-country skiing easily, once they learned to balance themselves with slippery five-feet boards on their feet.

But I had an edge, having skiied as a youth. While attending Carleton College in Minnesota, I occasionally worked out with the ski team during the winter before the start of indoor track. I went with them on cross-country tours. The captain of the ski team, John McCamant, conference 880 champion during the spring, tried to convince me I should join the squad full-time, and bridge the gap between cross-country running and skiing. I declined because of my lack of adaptability.

To compete on our college ski team, at least back in the 1950s, you had to partake in all four disciplines: downhill, slalom, ski jumping as well as cross-country skiing. If I could have specialized in just one, I might have competed. But it was a bit like a miler going out for track and being told he would have to pole vault, throw the discus and hurdle as well.

I enjoyed downhill skiing, however, and the things that went with downhill skiing (pretty girls). While in my early 20s, I made several pilgrimages to Aspen, Colo. The thrill of standing atop a mountain, then pushing off to slide down a trail of freshly fallen snow, leaving my mark on the mountainside, is still among my fonder memories. But from Aspen I also remember pushing myself too hard, catching an edge, tumbling and hearing something snap. Fortunately, it was my ski that broke, not my leg. But my knee was badly twisted. I finished my trip down the mountain aided by the Ski Patrol in a toboggan. Only after several days rest could I resume skiing.

The fear of that moment is still upon me even as I write this. You cannot ski successfully with fear. Part of my fear was that I would injure myself severely enough to interfere with my running interests, my Olympic ambitions. Back in that era, skiing and track seemed incompatible.

I am not so certain they are incompatible today, since cross-country skiing has advanced in popularity to the point where it almost has become a fad, like jogging a decade ago or bowling a decade before that. The boots and skis are lighter and better designed today. Back in the 1950s, I went cross-country skiing in downhill skis and boots, which is somewhat akin to wearing golf shoes for cross-country running.

As I glided through Bendix Woods, the sun sending shadows of trees across my path, I knew this experience would prove expensive. Because I was invigorated. I was having too much fun. Not this year, but probably next, I was going to have to equip myself with a set of cross-country skies, poles and boots—for a cost between $85 and $125. And I might wind up similarly equipping my wife and children at added expense. My 15-year-old daughter, Laura, already is into downhill skiing on rental equipment. It's always a good idea for fathers to relate to 15-year-old daughters.

(Skis cost $42.50; boots cost $32; bindings cost $8.50; poles cost $8.50. These are minimum costs, but thus equipped you can ski for free in many areas, unlike downhill skiing where travel and lift fees compromise even the amplest budgets.)

But then, as it happened with my venture into swimming, I discovered why I never became a champion skier. It occurred in an instant as I moved along a slope so gentle it was almost not a slope. Perhaps distracted by the scenery, my concentration lapsed. I allowed my weight to tilt backwards, a fatal flaw for any skier. Abruptly, my skis were out from under me and I landed flat on my back.

It was one of those jarring falls that on occasion can break bones. It knocked the breath from me. I lay dazed in the snow. My companion, Dick Gosswiller, first time ever on skis, who had been falling all afternoon but much less spectacularly, shouted,

"Are you all right?" I was, but it seemed possible that I might have just saved myself several hundred dollars.

No—I had so much fun that day, I'm still going to buy those cross-country skis.

I may also need to buy some equipment to enable me to play racquetball, since while researching this book I sampled that burgeoning sport also—and liked it.

My introduction to racquetball came several years previous while writing a book with Hank Stram, then coach of the Kansas City Chiefs. Stram loved the sport, and when Kansas City planned its multi-million-dollar football/baseball complex, somehow two racquetball courts found their way into construction plans. Stram played frequently, either at lunchtime or at the end of the day, dominated everybody he played against, including members of his football team, and claimed he never lost a game.

I watched several games from a door peephole, later sneaked onto one of the courts solo, learned I could hit the ball and eventually played several games with one of the equipment managers. (I lost.) On a trip to St. Louis the following winter, I visited my swimming neighbor, Sherman Atkinson, who had been transferred to that city by his employers, Midwest Steel. When I informed him of my impending visit, he announced we would have to play some racquetball, he and his wife Mary Ann recently having taken up the sport.

I was reluctant at first. I remembered them as tennis players. One winter Sherman, Mary Ann, my wife and I signed up for tennis lessons at the junior high school. It was an excuse to get out and do something at least one evening a week. I already knew how to play tennis and went along mainly to be sociable. I remembered Sherman and Mary Ann as the type of players for whom getting the ball over the net (much less into the right court) twice in a row would have been considered an accomplishment. And here they were challenging in racquetball an athlete trained on the courts of the Kansas City Chiefs!

Alas for my ego, the Atkinsons had been playing the game for nearly a year, several times a week. They had become, in fact, racquetball nuts, a breed kin to marathon nuts, tennis nuts, etc. On court with them on a Sunday morning, I suddenly found myself at their mercy. Balls came off the walls at me from all directions and all angles. I would move one way to reach a ball, and it would bounce the other way. They had me running up to the front wall, back to the rear wall, in both directions (sometimes at the same time) to the side walls.

They controlled my movements as might a puppetmaster his puppet. For a while, I stayed mildly competitive by running down each ball, but even the best-trained runner reaches his capacity after too many sprints. Before the end of our hour, I was totally exhausted; they seemed barely breathing hard.

Much later, while researching this book, I took several lessons. First, Chuck Sheftel, teaching pro at the Mid-Town Court House near downtown Chicago, and then Bonnie Korytowski, teaching at the Court House in Schaumburg near O'Hare Field, taught me the basics of the game.

Racquetball is an easy game to learn, Chuck explained, but a difficult game to master. Chuck taught tennis professionally for a dozen years before switching to racquetball, and he considered tennis much more difficult for beginners.

"Tennis takes a long time to learn," he claimed. "Initially, a beginner is picking up more balls than he is hitting. I could spend 10 weeks teaching someone tennis, and at the end he still might not be able to go out and play. But I can spend 10 minutes teaching racquetball, and I guarantee he can play the sport. They might not be able to play it well, but they can get out there, hit the ball and work up a sweat."

The advantage racquetball has over tennis is that its court is perhaps one-sixth the size. It also has four walls, and no matter which way you hit the ball, it bounces back to you. The racquet also is shorter, its handle chopped to half the length of a tennis racket, and therefore easier to handle. A tennis stroke must be made with a stiff forearm, but you snap your wrist when hitting a racquetball.

"It's a natural motion," explained Chuck, "somewhat like pitching a baseball."

But while racquetball can be learned easily, as Chuck explained, it is difficult to master, which may be part of its attraction. The game has many subtleties, as Bonnie explained to me during a second lesson.

"The player who controls the center of the court controls the game," she said, then demonstrated. Almost any ball hit off one of the side walls returns to the center. The person positioned there only needs patience to wait until it bounces to him to be able to hit it back. Balls hit straight off the wall can be reached by taking a step in either direction. The clever player tries to maneuver his opponent out of center court either by hitting the ball short to the wall or deep off the back wall. Racquetball is a fast-moving game where quick movements are essential, but it also is a game of strategy, and I could see myself becoming drawn to it.

It is possibly the fastest-growing sport in America in terms of popularity. In 1970, there were no racquetball court clubs in the United States and only 50,000 players, most of them persons who sneaked into handball courts to play, much to the displeasure of the handball players who claimed their racquets ruined the walls. By 1976, the figures had risen to 510 clubs and three million players. The number of balls sold from 1970 to 1976 rose from 228,000 to 10 million, another good index of the popularity of the sport.

The basic equipment for racquetball is inexpensive: a racquet costing $24, or $48 for the best models. Other than that, a player needs only a decent pair of tennis shoes, shorts, T-shirt and possibly a glove ($4.50). The continuing investment may be considerably higher. Yearly membership at the Court House in Chicago, for example, is $30, and court time costs $9 an hour, during the week, or $12 an hour in "prime time" (evenings and weekends). Playing the sport at the YMCA, however, may require less money—*if* you can reserve a court.

These figures are considerably less than for tennis. An inexpensive tennis racket costs about the same as a racquetball racquet of comparable quality, but top-grade tennis racquets may run as high as $185. Because indoor tennis courts require larger buildings with higher overhead, court fees also are higher: $12 to $16 an hour at Mid-Town Tennis Court in Chicago, owned by one of the owners of the Court House chain. Tennis players often dress more fashionably than racquetball players, who often appear wearing cutoffs. Where tennis becomes somewhat less expensive for long-range play is when warm weather beckons, play being free on most outdoor courts—if you can find one empty. If not, you may have to swallow the expense of country club membership where you can reserve courts in advance.

If tennis has a flaw as a sport, it is not cost or difficulty but this country club image, which has only begun to diminish in the last decade as the sport's basic attractiveness has been discovered by more and more people.

I once profiled Billie Jean King for the *New York Times Magazine*, and she told me, "If tennis ever is going anywhere, we need to get more ordinary people involved." If anyone succeeded in doing that, it was Billie Jean, who learned the sport playing on public courts. Even more than any male tennis player in the last several decades, she has been the most exciting tennis personality.

Recently, I renewed my acquaintance with tennis, because my 16-year-old son, David, began playing the game. It is always good for fathers to relate to 16-year-old sons. He lettered as a freshman in high school and was elected captain of the team in 1976, his sophomore year, winning a majority of his matches.

I'm not sure where he got his talent, because I was merely adequate as a tennis player while growing up. I do remember some stirring matches I played with Paul Baptist, who pole vaulted and ran the two-mile on our track team, while attending graduate school at the University of Chicago. During the summer of 1954, we often played once or twice a week.

I still remember one morning when a three-set match between us lasted four hours. This was before tie-breakers, and each set lasted forever. Most games were deuce games. Most points involved long rallies. The margin of victory in games, after four hours, was 31-29. It was stunning tennis, the way the game should be played, not because either of us was any good, but because we were evenly matched.

This was the main problem I faced when, several years ago, in a year away from running competition, I attempted to reinvolve myself with tennis. After several practice matches with friends who were either too good for me or not good enough, I entered a local tournament, hoping to find others on my level, and got shut out, 6-0, 6-0, in the first round. I tried again and once more lost, 6-0, 6-0.

It was not that I minded losing, except that in examining the result sheets I could see other opening-round players also getting shut out by similar scores. The way tennis is scored and played, it often is easy for a player to skunk someone just one level below him. In the method of seeding tournaments, top-ranked players are sprinkled evenly through the draw so as not to eliminate each other immediately. So what happens is they eliminate lesser players immediately. Were there a second or third round for losers, these lesser players might at least encounter someone of equal ability (or equal lack of it). Instead, the losers go home and wait for the next tournament—or perhaps decide against entering any more.

That was the case with me, because I put away my tennis racket midway through the summer and went back to running where beginning joggers seem to be welcomed with much more sympathy. On the other hand, had I the patience to persevere in tennis, I eventually might have found another "Paul Baptist."

I had more success when I moved into cycling as a sport. I still have not attempted a competitive race as a cyclist, so I avoided the mistake I made in tennis. But I have taken several long touring trips.

The main appeal of cycling is you can just do it. You do not need fancy equipment: either on your back or under your seat. The simplest thing in the world is to grab a bike out of the back shed and pedal off down the road. My wife, Rose, enjoys cycling, so frequently on summer evenings, we go for a ride along the lakeshore for three or four miles. It is a good idea for a father to relate to the mother of his children.

Once you get involved in the sport, however, you may want to buy a 10-speed bicycle (instead of merely a "bike"), and although discount stores will sell you one for less than $100, you also can spend as much today for a bicycle ($800) as people two generations ago spent for new automobiles. As I write this, I am planning to buy an exercise cycle (cost $125) for my wife to use indoors during the winter.

The person who talked me into doing some serious bicycling was Edwin C. Johnson, a management consultant and executive recruiter from Chicago. I got to know Ed in the mid-1960s while writing a book on consulting entitled *The Business Healers*. We became close friends. Ed played squash, handball, tennis, skied, scuba-dived and cycled. He was my picture of what an active man should be.

One summer, we invited Ed and his wife, Tish, to Long Beach for the day and asked them to bring their bicycles. Our whole family cycled with them seven or eight miles along some back roads to a nearby small town called New Buffalo, had a beer (Coke for the kids), then cycled back. At the end of the day, Ed asked me for $5, accepted the money and told me I had just purchased his 10-speed Rudge. He had just bought a new Cinelli. His old model was somewhat battered but a bargain at any price less than $150.

I think he wanted to get me interested in bicycle racing, figuring that my distance runner's endurance would make me competitive in that sport, too. Perhaps I could bridge the gap between road racing and road cycling, but not being mechanically inclined, I have little interest in the maintenance necessary for success as a serious cycler. My idea of how to fix a flat tire is, you pile your bike in the back of your car and take it to a bike shop. Ed fixes his flats where they happen. Also, to be truly competitive as a cyclist, you have to be into such things as boiling your chain in hot water the night before the race then coating it with wax.

Eventually, Ed Johnson talked me into making a three-day bike trip over one Labor Day weekend with him and a Chicago attorney named Ed Roth. We planned to fly with our bicycles to Ashland, Wisc., then follow a carefully prepared route along back roads to La Crosse, Wisc., a distance of more than 200 miles.

The trip was fraught with problems. We lost half a day's cycling when I bent a wheel hitting a pothole at night. Ed Johnson had similar trouble, and had to stay up most of the night and part of the next day making repairs before hitching a ride to catch us. Thus delayed, we found ourselves on the third day far from our destination, bucking 30-40 m.p.h. headwinds. Eventually, we stopped short. But it had been a thrilling experience. I came away from the trip feeling a sense of accomplishment, as though I had climbed a high mountain or finished the Boston Marathon.

Cycling does have its own Boston Marathon, but it is not a race. It is the Tour of the Scioto River Valley (better known as TOSRV) held the Mother's Day weekend each May. It is strictly for touring cyclists who gather in Columbus, Ohio, Friday night, spend all day Saturday cycling 115 miles south to a small Ohio River town called Portsmouth, then spend all Sunday cycling back north along a slightly shorter course. Each year, 3400—and no more than 3400—cyclists take part in the touring event. It is first come, first served, and anyone wishing to enter TOSRV must return applications within a few days after official entry forms go out each January.

Unlike Boston, there is no single start from a specific starting line at a particular time. Cyclists simply roll out of their motel rooms early in the morning and head down the road in great masses. The pace for most is casual, friendly, but every so often a group of serious racers rushes past, single-file, wheel-on-wheel, drafting each other for maximum speed. I found it fun, on occasion, to fall into the draft and sprint down the highway at top speed. At several rest points, we stopped for sandwiches and drinks, supplied by organizers. Unlike our Wisconsin tour, where we carried packs on our bikes, we had no gear to worry about, that being transported for us by "sag-wagons."

En route back to Columbus the next morning, we pedaled several hours through a drenching rainstorm. Being used to running in all types of weather, it did not bother me. The sun came out and warmed us toward the end of our trip. I had a flat, and Ed Johnson cursed my incompetence in changing it, then did the job for me. If you want to take long tours, it helps to have someone like him along.

At the end of the day in Columbus, we received fancy patches and richly colored certificates announcing our achievements in finishing TOSRV. Ed said a lot of cyclists would love to have that certificate. But instead of framing it, I tucked it away in some drawer when I got home. The achievement was in having done it. I have certificates from the Boston Marathon (I have run the race 10 times), which I never bothered to frame, either, although the trophy I won for placing fifth in that race one year is prominently displayed in the living room.

TOSRV is but one of many cycling tours available in all parts of the United States. They vary in distance from a few miles to the length of the country itself. Increasing numbers of bike paths are appearing throughout the United States. The Calumet Bikeway, a nine-mile-long crushed gravel trail, opened recently in the Dunes National Lakeshore not far from our home. My wife and I traveled over it one weekend last fall.

But swimming, skiing, racquetball, tennis, cycling and any other sports that from time to time catch my fancy probably will never be more than merely temporary diversions. I like to run. I have an 18-year-old son, Kevin, who competes in track. He is one of Indiana's top high school distance runners and placed fifth in the state cross-country championship his senior year. In workouts now, he already beats me. I train often with him, because it's a good idea for a father to relate to his 18-year-old son.

Running is what I do best. It is fun for me. When I am in top condition, there are very few people in the world in my age division capable of beating me. Fortunately, I have chosen a sport which is not only one of the least expensive of those previously mentioned (the basic cost is a pair of $25 running shoes), but also one in which maximum physical benefits can be received.

But while the best sport for me is running, it may not necessarily be the best sport for everyone. What is the best sport for you? Let us consider that question in the next chapter.

13

The Pain of P.E.

One of the greatest myths perpetrated on the American public over the last four decades has been the notion that exercise or physical activity is not fun. Perhaps the myth has been with us even longer, but I have only been around that long. A second sub-myth is that you need to make exercise fun in order to get people to do it.

Well, I suppose that depends on your definition of fun. To me, running is fun. For others, it is not. Although I would find pressing my body weight overhead practically impossible, I also rather enjoy weight lifting when I occasionally do it. Perhaps it is the discipline involved that appeals to me.

Various means have evolved as to how you can sugar-coat exercise. When I watched Barry Franklin's exercise regimen in Cleveland, he had a group of older men lying in a circle on the ground pushing a medicine ball back and forth in the air with their feet as an alternative to doing sit-ups. Personally, I would rather do the sit-ups, but that is my nature. If utilization of a medicine ball, or any other gimmick, inspires someone else to get in shape or stay in shape, fine!

But I sometimes wonder if the general public's reaction to exercise is partly a conditioned response. We think exercise is not fun, because over the years we have been taught and told it is not fun. In some respect, Barry Franklin's fine program, which he borrowed from his teacher at Penn State, Karl G. Stoedefalke, is a denial of the fact that fitness can be enjoyable for its own sake.

This gets back to the conditioning factor. For example, my daughter Laura played on her junior high school volleyball team last winter. If you asked the average person whether or not he considered volleyball a fun sport, he probably would say yes. It is a game played with a ball. Games played with balls are fun; so goes the conditioned response.

Volleyball is a game played with a community of people; it is a team sport. Unless you play at the Olympic level, where competitors dive at the floor for balls, little pain is involved. You can get mildly out of breath. You can burn calories. You can have a good time.

In fact, Barry Franklin suggests that older people play a variation on the sport where one bounce of the ball on the ground is permitted, in addition to three hits in the air, before it has to be hit over the net. "You get longer rallies that way," he explains, "and it doesn't require as high a skill level to get something out of the sport." He is probably right.

During the summer of 1976, when I served as a guest lecturer at Runner's Mecca, the high-altitude running camp in Utah, we played volleyball as a diversion between long-distance runs. We often played in combination with some of Marc Sorenson's dieters from the National Institute of Fitness. No one forced us to play volleyball. It was fun.

But my daughter's volleyball coach forced her and other members of the team to run. It was done in this manner. After Laura or one of the other members of the team made an error, the coach said, "That's one more lap you have to run." At the end of practice, the girls ran laps around the gym as a form of punishment. The coach was conditioning them to believe that while volleyball may be fun, running is not.

That coach was not alone in using running—whether laps

around a gym or wind sprints—as a form of punishment. With that sort of message coming down from our physical education instructors, is it any wonder that the rate of deaths from heart attacks in the United States is so high?

When we start talking about running as a punishment, however, it reminds me of a discussion I had with Rich Stolbach, a teacher from Tarrytown, N.Y., who was part of our group at Runner's Mecca. During an evening when Marc Sorenson talked to us about diet, Rick described some difficulties he had at school.

Apparently, he was giving a party for the children in his class, and he refused to buy candy bars for them as did all the other teachers whenever they offered parties. Eventually, he had to appear before a grievance committee hearing to explain his actions.

"Whenever we have a party at school, we always hand out candy and cookies," Rick explained. "So what we do is we condition children to associate pleasant conditions with poor nutrition."

And in the meantime, we punish them by making them run in the gym!

Even track coaches often use running as a form of punishment. In the early 1960s, a former classmate from Mt. Carmel High School in Chicago, Fred Weber, asked me to help him coach the track team. When we were in school together, Fred played starting halfback on a very good football team and ran the sprints in track. Unfortunately, he brought some of his football exercises with him to our cross-country workouts. One such exercise was to have the cross-country team members poise in the push-up position, then release their arms and crash to the ground.

I eventually steered him away from that exercise, since most distance runners have less padding on their bodies than their counterparts in football. But as I look back on some of the alternative exercises I proposed, they were not much better. As recently as a decade ago, most track runners (myself included) used calisthenics as a means of warming up for workouts. Today, calisthenics is out; yoga is in. Stretching exercises are considered a better means of preparation. And you no longer bounce up and down vigorously to touch your toes; you str-e-e-e-tch and reach down slowly to grasp them.

But one thing Fred and I did right in coaching our team was that we used running as a reward rather than as a punishment. The better runners were allowed to run more, because they were better runners. It was an honor to take extra laps in practice. The top runner on our squad was Bill Hoffmann, who won city championships in track and cross-country. He set the standard for the team.

We did a lot of "interval" training in that era, and I might have Bill run six or eight laps of around 1000 yards around the perimeter of our workout area in the park. In between, he would rest briefly, jogging or walking. Various other members of the team did fewer laps, depending on their ability. Some runners might do two loops with Bill, then rest one before rejoining him again. Others might run every other one. Still others might run one and rest two. I gauged each person's ability to continue according to how tired he looked running the previous one. So being able to do more running, rather than less, became a status symbol on our team.

I recall one day during the track season when Bill was doing a workout consisting of 16 440s on the track, jogging an equal distance between each one. He ran them at a pace around 70 seconds per quarter-mile. At the beginning, all the distance runners ran with Bill. As each of them reached his limit at that pace—four 440s, six, eight, sometimes walking instead of jogging between—I permitted them to leave practice early.

Soon, there remained only two runners: Bill and George Yergans, the latter a tall, skinny black athlete who also high jumped well enough to place in several of our meets but who had not broken five minutes for a mile the previous year. George began to exhibit signs of fatigue, so midway through the workout I told him he was excused from practice. But no, he wanted to continue. He would fall behind during the jogging lap between 440s, then would cut across the infield to be ready for the start of the next one. I kept asking him if he had enough, but he still wanted to keep going. Soon, he was down to walking between 440s, and in the last few he simply waited at the line for the next to begin. But he ran all 16 of the 440s, and it was obvious from the look on his face that he felt he had achieved a personal victory.

At the city championships later that spring, Bill Hoffmann

placed second in the mile with 4:27, an excellent performance for him as a junior; he would win that race the following year. George Yergans, then a senior, placed fifth in that race with 4:36, an astounding improvement of his personal best. I only coached a few years at Mt. Carmel, but when I look back on my achievements, I rate George Yergans' fifth place as the greatest. Of course, it actually was his achievement, not mine.

To fully assess my success as a teacher, however, you would have to locate all the members of that team and determine how many of them still are running—or participating in other forms of physical fitness. I know of at least one (Ernie Harris, a former half-miler), but I hope there are others.

I have other memories of my own days in high school, not all of them pleasant. Carmel, an all-boys school, had 1000 students and (as far as I can remember) one gym teacher, who shall go nameless here. I remember him as always wearing a white T-shirt, having a crewcut that was almost a shaved head and carrying a belt in his hand, since he used it as a weapon to keep boys in line. Well, we needed some form of discipline. With between 150 and 200 boys in a single class, and only one instructor, what else could you do?

I remember each class as a madhouse with us doing one type of calisthenic after another—or *not* doing them, since the most-often-played game was loafing when the gym teacher looked the other way. We spent more energy trying to avoid exercise then we would have doing it.

An even-more-favored game was getting (or sometimes even forging) a doctor's excuse saying you could not participate in strenuous exercise. That meant you could sit in the bleachers and either do your homework or snicker at those forced to exercise. I often took the doctor's excuse route—*I*, the one who is now writing a book about physical fitness! One of the motivating factors that got me out for track was that if you were member of a varsity team, you did not have to take gym. Mt. Carmel, partly as a result, had very strong varsity sports.

That instructor, God love him, is now dead. But how many boys did he teach to hate physical activity? Occasionally, I attend the annual reunions of my former high school where I notice an overabundance of bellies overlapping belts. And yet, when you mention that former gym instructor's name, everyone gets misty-eyed and speaks of him with reverence.

I also sometimes attend reunions for the college I attended: Carleton College in Northfield, Minn. Recently, at our class's 20th reunion, I was surprised by the number who approached me to announce they were into running. Without having kept score, I guess there were maybe as many as six, an impressive number when you consider our graduating class was only 200 and most were not at the reunion. One former classmate, Chuck Cranston, lived in Alaska and often ran distances of eight or 10 miles.

One embryo jogger was Dave Sipfle, now a department chairman at my alma mater. I remembered Dave as being almost the antithesis of the athlete during his college days. If you were taking a vote as to the person least likely to succeed in any form of sports, it would most likely have been Dave.

He admitted as much to me when he said, "I never even knew I had a body until I was 30 years old." Now he is into tennis, squash, cross-country skiing and who knows what else?

I don't know the answer, but I can't help but wonder whether or not there are certain basic flaws in the physical education programs in the United States that cause the Dave Sipfles to have to wait so long to discover their bodies.

14
What Sports Are Best for Fitness?

Assuming we agree that exercise is good for you, the question now is: How much exercise? And what kind of exercise? Until Kenneth H. Cooper, M.D., wrote *Aerobics*, nobody had been able to demonstrate successfully, with any scientific precision, how much exercise to take. It all depended on the individual. And even Dr. Cooper's tables and point charts are only suggestions as to how much you should exercise. He has good data supporting his contention that someone earning 30-34 points can significantly reduce their chances of having a heart attack. But some people, depending on their personal habits, probably can do less. And others may want to do more.

It all depends on the individual. What is too much for some people would be too little for others. The amount of exercise should in part depend on your desire. In no sense should you take exercise as you might medicine.

According to Wes McVicar, national director of physical education for the YMCA in Canada, "One should be able to develop a philosophy which permits you to play not because it is beneficial, but because one likes to do it. This means that play itself should not be taken too seriously; otherwise, one form of tension is merely substituted for another."

Nevertheless, it helps to have a goal. Having some ends in mind can help motivate you to exercise. Perhaps you want to swim a mile non-stop, or run a mile in six minutes, or you want to beat a certain racquetball player at your club. Such goals can help spur you on. But do not set a goal too high; otherwise, you may become discouraged at your failure to approach it. Leave the world records for members of the Olympic team.

What sort of exercise is best for you? In other words, what sports are best for fitness?

The best sport is the one you enjoy, because you will probably be more faithful in sticking to it. Regularity in any sport provides the best success. It's better to exercise easily once a day, or two or three times a week, than to exercise strenuously on a hit-and-miss basis.

Warren Guild, M.D., once said, "It is easy to predict when a weekend athlete will die. He will die on a weekend."

While picking a sport you like, you should give some thought to available facilities. If you are near a lake or a pool, it might be most convenient to take up swimming. If tennis courts or ice skating ponds are nearby, you might want to take up those sports. You could build yourself a gym in your basement, complete with exercise cycle and weight lifting equipment.

But in addition to convenience, think of enjoyment. Even if you live right next to a lake, you might still rather travel 10 miles to the nearest racquetball court if you dislike getting wet.

Some sports, however, will do a better job than others in improving your physical fitness and in helping you resist the familiar danger discussed so frequently in the pages of this book: the heart attack that each year kills 600,000 Americans.

Until recently, physiologists could only make educated guesses as to the best fitness exercises, then along came individuals like Dr. Cooper with scientific results to prove or disprove those guesses. Dr. Cooper's Aerobics points are one means of determining whether or not a certain activity results in fitness. Another measurement is the number of "mets" (see Chapter 5) that activity requires. Still another measurement is the number of calories the activity burns. (Chapter 10.) And somewhere in the formula should be some consideration as to whether or not the activity is interesting (i.e., "fun") or dangerous.

In this chapter, I have attempted to rate different sports, or forms of exercise, the way a movie critic might rate a motion picture: four stars for those providing the best route to fitness to zero stars for those providing no fitness benefits. While there was no absolute standard that separated one level from another, in order to earn four-star rating a sport needed to provide a minimum of 15 Aerobics points per hour, provide five mets in terms of energy expenditure and burn at least 500 calories per hour.*

It should also be moderately enjoyable and relatively risk-free. All the four-star sports in the following ratings meet that standard, but I confess I realized this only *after* I rated them, not before. A certain amount of educated guessing still was necessary.

Meaning of the ratings

* * * *	Excellent form of exercise; provides maximum fitness.
* * *	Good form of exercise; provides reasonable amount of fitness.
* *	Fair form of exercise; provides moderate amount of fitness.
*	Poor form of exercise; provides minimal amount of fitness.
zero	Provides no fitness benefits.

---

* My source for Aerobics points was *Aerobics* by Kenneth H. Cooper, M.D. The met table (approximate metabolic cost of activities) came from *Modern Concepts of Cardiovascular Disease* by S.M. Fox, J.P. Naughton and P.A. Gorman. The calorie table used is from one prepared by Robert E. Johnson, M.D., and colleagues at the University of Illinois and presented in a booklet by the American Medical Association entitled, *Basic Bodywork...for Fitness and Health*. They were computed for an individual weighing 150 pounds.

1. RUNNING

Pros: Without question, running ranks as the most efficient form of exercise. If you are exercising according to Dr. Cooper's Aerobics program, you can earn more points in less time by becoming a runner.* According to Dr. Cooper, "You definitely get more benefit—and quicker—from running than any other form of exercise. Look at the examples: five points in eight minutes! You get more benefit from this than you do from seven hours of golf!"

If you are interested in losing weight, no other activity beats running. According to tables prepared by Robert E. Johnson, M.D., of the University of Illinois, by running at 10 miles per hour you can burn 900 calories during that period of time (90 calories per mile). No other activity measured by Dr. Johnson and his colleagues in the Department of Physiology and Biophysics came even close, except scull rowing in a race (840 points). Even the beginning jogger who plods along at an easy 12 minutes per mile (five m.p.h.) pace burns calories at a rate of 450 per hour. The 10 m.p.h. runner is exercising at the 17-met level; the 5 m.p.h. jogger, 7-8 mets.

Running also benefits every muscle group in the body, tones the arms, trims the stomach. But its most important benefit is cardiovascular. According to physiologist David L. Costill of the Human Performance Laboratory at Ball State University, "In order to metabolize excessive fats from your blood stream, you need to do your exercise at relatively low intensity and for a long period of time. That's why nothing can equal running, or long-course swimming, or continous cycling for benefitting your heart."

But perhaps one of the biggest arguments in favor of running is its basic simplicity. Barring some physical handicap, anybody can do it. It takes no talent, ability or specific coordination. The graceless plodder can achieve the same physiological benefits as the Olympic athlete.

Running is an inexpensive sport: no special equipment is needed except possibly a very good pair of shoes. You need no costly club memberships, since you can jog around the block. You

---

* For practical considerations, running and jogging are the same activity; jogging is simply slow running. The difference between runners and joggers is mostly state of mind.

need not find a partner or recruit enough people to form two or more teams.

Provided proper precautions are taken, running can be done in all forms of weather including pouring rainstorms and blizzards. I have run without ill effects on icy streets around my home with a wind-chill factor of 67 degrees below zero and on the streets near my brother-in-law's home in Mesa, Ariz., when the temperature was 112 degrees. I admittedly was not running very fast either time, but I was running.

It is also an exercise that can be continued all your life. "What I like about running most," says Dr. Cooper, "is that I can recommend it to anyone of any age." Amos Alonzo Stagg, the former famous University of Chicago football coach, played tennis until age 83, then switched to running. He continued to jog in his back yard until age 96, when the cataracts in his eyes became so bad he began bumping into trees. Larry Lewis, a waiter from San Francisco, continued running 100-yard sprints until he died at age 104.

Cons: Running can strain the joints of the body, particularly if done on hard roads, on too-small indoor tracks (or around basketball courts), in poorly fitting, worn-down shoes or with excessive zeal.

The parts of the body most likely to suffer injury are the knees, ankles and achilles tendons. If the type of running includes all-out sprinting, muscle tears may result.

It is also a less satisfactory sport for heavily-muscled individuals who become frustrated when persons, whose faces they once kicked sand into at the beach, speed past them. By running, you probably will become lean and hungry, losing that cherubic look that many American mothers (incorrectly) associate with good health. Women runners also will discover that as they continue to run, their waistline will shrink, but so may their bra size.

Perhaps the most poignant criticism of running comes from people who state, "It just isn't fun." Although the boredom factor in running can be alleviated partially by seeking new running areas and training with companions, there is no easy solution for a person who takes that point of view.

Aerobics points per hour	60 (10 m.p.h.)
Calories burned per hour	900 (10 m.p.h.)
	726 (6 m.p.h.)
Mets	17 (10 m.p.h.)
	10 (6 m.p.h.)
Interest level	fair
Injury risk level	low
Rating	* * * *

2. SWIMMING

Pros: Almost all of the positive things said about running can also be said about swimming. Dr. Cooper rates it a close second to running when he compares exercises for their ability to provide physical fitness. Cooper states, "The big advantage of swimming is that, for most people, it is much more enjoyable than running. There is a social atmosphere around a pool you won't find on a track at six in the morning."

And Dr. Ransom J. Arthur adds, "There is a rhythmical sensation in swimming not dissimilar to that of dancing, and there is the pleasant feel of the water enveloping and soothing the entire body."

If you are interested in body strength, swimming exercises the shoulders more than almost any other sport besides weight lifting, and it also strengthens the legs.

The cost of equipment (one bathing suit) is less than that for any other sport, although membership in a YMCA or sports club, in order to have access to facilities, may raise the cost of participation somewhat.

Swimming, like running, also has the advantage of being a sport that requires no partners.

David L. Costill (who once swam competitively for Ohio University, placing third in the nationals one year in the butterfly stroke) considers swimming an excellent activity—although still second to running, which he now does. It meets his criteria (in metabolizing fats from the bloodstream) for being an exercise that can be done at a relatively low intensity for a long period of time.

But perhaps the greatest advantage swimming has over any

sport is that, excluding the fact that you can drown in a pool or a lake, you face much less risk of injury than in almost any sport.

According to Dr. Arthur, "No other physical activity offers such an unlimited possibility of exercise without the dangers inherent in body contact sports, or the joint, bone and muscle problems that plague runners, tennis players and gymnasts. The water of a pool supports the body and inflicts no jarring pressures on the joints."

In terms of comparing the efficiency of swimming, in both weight loss and cardiovascular activity, it is difficult to make a precise decision on the basis of figures available. According to Dr. Cooper, a swimmer who covers 600 yards (24 laps in most pools) between 10 and 15 minutes earns five points. It should take him twice as long as a runner moving at average speed to earn the same number of points.

Dr. Johnson identified swimming as burning only 300 calories per hour compared to 900 for running, but measured swimming at one-fourth m.p.h., a relatively gentle pace compared to the 10 m.p.h. at which he measured runners. Comparable effort for swimmers probably would result in the calorie loss of at least 600, but it would depend partly on the efficiency of the swimmers involved.

Physiologists have neglected swimmers in the laboratory, because it is much more difficult to measure them during exercise. You cannot, using present technology, monitor a swimmer with an electrocardiograph or collect oxygen samples. Were this possible, researchers might discover that swimming, with an equal expenditure of energy, is every bit as efficient as running in terms of both cardiovascular benefits and weight reduction.

Cons: You cannot carry a swimming pool in your gym bag as you can a pair of running shoes. You need a pool, or at least a body of water such as a lake or an ocean, to exercise. If your choice of locale is only the latter, you may have to find some other activity during cold-weather months. If you catch colds easily, or are bothered by chlorine, swimming may not appeal to you. As with running, boredom also may be a factor, particularly in 25-yard pools where the swimmer must go up and back, up and back.

Swimming probably is a less satisfactory activity for skinny individuals, those persons who after having sand kicked in their faces at the beach took up running despite Charles Atlas' pleas. Because they lack body bulk, they also lack buoyancy. The competitive sport of swimming also concentrates more on short-distance events than the long-distance events which are so popular (and more beneficial) in running. Swimming the English Channel, unfortunately, will never have the mass attraction for participants as running the Boston Marathon.

Aerobics points per hour	15 (1 m.p.h.)
Calories burned per hour	600 (0.5 m.p.h.)
Mets	no rating available
Interest level	fair
Injury risk level	extremely low
Rating	* * * *

3. CYCLING

Pros: Anyone who considers running a boring activity or who dislikes jumping into a swimming pool can probably achieve an equal level of fitness by climbing on a bicycle and pedaling down the road.

Dr. Cooper considers cycling "a good match for running and swimming." He adds, "The aerobic benefits—the training effect—to the internal organs are identical with those of running and swimming."

David L. Costill agrees and says that cycling also meets his criteria for a low-intensity, long-level exercise that seems to metabolize fat rapidly. He cautions, however, that in order to obtain the proper benefits cycling must be continuous, "not where you glide all over the place."

Both Cooper and Costill further indicate that equal benefit can be obtained from a stationary, indoor exercise bicycle—as long as *you* supply the power.

Cycling at eight m.p.h. uses 5-6 mets. Speeding up to 13 m.p.h. uses 8-9 mets.

In terms of Aerobics points, a cyclist who covers 20 miles an hour (very fast, and probably the equivalent in energy spent to a runner who goes 10 miles in that time) earns 20 points. In terms of weight reduction, Dr. Johnson rates cycling at 13 m.p.h. (a more reasonable pace, but still fast) as burning 660 calories, third on his charts only to running and scull racing.

If you are not interested in speed, cycling is relatively inexpensive. A reasonably good multi-speed bicycle can be purchased for probably less than would cost a year's membership in a health club, such as the YMCA. You not only do not need a partner to go cycling, but if you want one you probably will have less difficulty recruiting one than for running or swimming.

Probably the greatest attraction of cycling is that it permits you, even *compels* you, to get out and enjoy the scenery. This same benefit is available to competitive runners, who through their ability cover distances of 10-20 miles daily in training get a chance to sightsee while they work out. The average YMCA jogger's equivalent in cycling, however, can cover three or four times the distance with relatively little strain and see much more scenery. He also can dismount and enjoy a particular spot much more easily than the runner whose activity must be more or less continuous from start to finish. (The same with swimmers, who sink if they stop swimming.)

An even greater plus for serious cyclists are the availability of an increasing number of touring events sponsored by local bicycle groups affiliated with the League of American Wheelmen. On weekends, they often travel in groups for distances from 25 to several hundred miles. The cyclists thus are able to achieve the best of both worlds: they obtain the camaraderie that distance runners find at events such as the Boston Marathon without the excessive stress present in competition.

Cons: You need to buy a bicycle and while, admittedly, a basic bike is relatively expensive, a 10-speed foreign model can cost as much as $800. Bicycles also have flat tires (something that never happens to runners or swimmers), and this can be either a nuisance or a serious problem, depending on how adept you are at fixing flats or how far away from home it occurs.

Another problem that cyclists and swimmers share is that in certain parts of the country weather limits the season. While a few dedicated cyclists bundle up and bike in the coldest temperatures, even they are helpless when faced by icy roads.

Cycling also does not exercise all parts of the body as well as swimming or, particularly, running. "Cycling is limited because it isolates the thighs," admits David Costill. And Dr. Cooper explains, "Most of the power is supplied by the hips and legs, and consequently most of the toughening up goes to these areas."

Although the risk of muscle injury to recreational cyclists is almost non-existent, cyclists who insist on racing at high speeds can seriously injure themselves if they fall off, one reason why they wear protective headgear. Recreational cyclists sometimes also get moving at high speeds, particularly going downhill, and if they fall off they are less likely to have headgear for protection.

But perhaps an even greater hazard for cyclists is that frequently they must share road space with automobiles, which have greater mass and travel at greater velocity. In a collision between a motorist and a cyclist, only the latter gets hurt. This hazard recently has been lessened somewhat by the development of more bike trails and bike lanes on city streets, but the number of cyclists (and motorists) increases the likeliness of accidents.

Aerobics points per hour	20 (20 m.p.h.)
Calories burned per hour	660 (13 m.p.h.)
Mets	8-9 (13 m.p.h.)
Interest level	high
Injury risk level	very low to very high
Rating	* * * *

4. CROSS-COUNTRY SKIING

Pros: The popularity of this sport only became apparent midway through this decade. In fact, the boom in cross-country skiing probably only has begun. When Dr. Cooper published *Aerobics* in 1968, he failed to mention cross-country skiing on a list of "additional exercises" that included fencing, rope skipping and lacrosse. He did include "skiing" (snow or water) and suggested that an hour of activity in these sports (which actually are quite dissimilar) would earn you six points. An asterisk referred readers to the bottom of the page where they learned they only received that point level if their activity was continuous—and few mountains are long enough to permit continuous downhill skiing. Dr. Cooper would probably be the first to admit that his points rating for skiing represented, at best, an educated guess.

By the time Dr. Cooper published *The New Aerobics* in 1970, he had awakened to the potential of cross-country (as opposed to downhill skiing). "Triple the value," he suggested, meaning that an hour of cross-country skiing earned the participant 18 points. If anything, Dr. Cooper probably was being conservative. If a cross-country skier pursued his activity at the same energy level as a runner, he probably would equal the runner's capacity (at six-minute mile pace) to score 60 Aerobics points in an hour.

Dr. Johnson rates the energy expenditure of skiing at 10 m.p.h. at 600 calories. Ski touring at 5 m.p.h. in loose snow costs 10 mets.

David L. Costill, who often goes cross-country skiing for periods up to an hour and a half when enough snow falls near his home in Muncie, Ind., ranks the sport as equal to running and swimming. "In terms of fat metabolism, it's probably better," Costill suggests. "It also does much more for the body musculature. The advantage cross-country skiing has over jogging is that you use your upper body more."

When it comes to cost, cross-country skiing falls somewhere in the middle ground between the very cheap exercises (running, swimming) and the very expensive exercises, which would include downhill skiing. A set of skis, boots, bindings and poles come in between $85 and $125 according to my local ski shop in Michigan City, Ind.: A Bit of Scandinavia. The added cost of skiing, however, increases in relation to your own fashion-consciousness, but this is true of running and cycling as well.

A major advantage of the sport of cross-country skiing is that if you enjoy scenery, you can get out into areas you never would see driving along the highway in a car. And although the sport can be pursued aggressively (like running), it also can be approached gently (like jogging). The variety of experiences available on cross-country skis (which includes some downhill skiing as well) makes for a very low boredom level.

Cons: Snow. Unless you have it, you're shut out. Obviously, cross-country skiing is a much easier activity to engage in for residents of Minnesota than for residents of Florida. Also, it takes more organization than many other sports, since skis must be waxed and sometimes packed in, or on, a car so you can travel to a suitable area for ski touring. Because of the logistics problems, most people will find it difficult to engage in the sport much more often than on weekends, suggesting that they could benefit from an alternate mid-week sport such as running or swimming.

(Bonnie Korytowski, a racquetball instructor for the Court House in Schaumberg, Ill., told me she was so eager to go cross-country skiing that, when the first snow fell during the winter of 1976, she went out back of her apartment and skied up and down the alley. One homeowner was shovelling the area behind his garage, and she pleaded with him to finish the job later. Being a gentleman, he obliged.)

One negative factor is that skiing is a technique sport. It requires at least average coordination and fairly good balance if you do not want to spend all your time picking yourself up out of the snow. If God had wanted man to walk with six-foot boards on his feet, he would have given him size 60 feet. Balancing on smoothly waxed skis on slippery snow presents problems, particularly going up and down hills. Lessons from a competent professional are necessary for even the most talented athletes. It is a sport in which part of the beauty is being able to skim smoothly across the snow in almost ballet-like movements. Whereas an individual with poor running technique will persevere as a jogger, a skier who keeps falling will soon find another sport.

The risk of injury, while nowhere near as great as in downhill skiing, also is a factor in cross-country skiing. Ankles can be twisted, knees can be wrenched, muscles can be torn, and legs can be broken even by competent skiers.

Aerobics points per hour	18*
Calories burned per hour	600 (10 m.p.h.)
Mets	10 (5 m.p.h., loose snow)
Interest level	good
Injury risk level	medium
Rating	* * * *

5. WALKING

Pros: Probably the least demanding of all exercises is simply putting on a comfortable pair of shoes, opening your front door and going for a long walk. It is a form of exercise that can be engaged in by people of all ages, of all body types and of all levels of coordination. For those people at a low fitness level, it is the activity you begin before you start more vigorous sports. For those people who grade in his Fitness Category I (very poor), Dr. Cooper recommends three weeks of walking before taking the first jogging step. He blends three more weeks of walking and jogging before permitting them to run as far as a mile.

* Estimated.

Despite its simplicity, walking promises enormous benefits, especially if it is coupled with a regular program of calisthenic-type exercises. Provided you wear the right clothing, you can walk in all sorts of weather, including rain and snowstorms. And by taking the time to look around while you walk, you can see things you would completely miss travelling by car (or swimming in a pool at the YMCA).

Since walking is the least demanding of all exercises, it can be done by people of all ages. One of Dr. Paul Dudley White's patients came in for a checkup at age 102 and was advised to continue walking his customary mile a day. He lived to be 107. Mrs. Emma Gatewood of Gallipolis, Ohio, was 69 when she walked from Oglethorpe, Ga., to Mount Katahidin, Maine, a distance of 1500 miles. An Arab named Touat Mohand Said walked 93 miles to Algiers at the age of 109 to claim his pension.

If you want to increase the level of stress, you can walk with a pack on your back or in rough, hilly backwoods areas. Walking up very steep hills is known as mountain climbing. Unless you progress to this level in your hikes, the risk of injury is very slight.

David L. Costill states, "If you walk about three miles a day, which takes about an hour, then you probably develop pretty good muscle and metabolize a lot of fat."

In terms of weight reduction, walking burns off body fat at the same rate as running: 90 calories per mile. Long-distance runners often are horrified and outraged when someone informs them of this fact, but it is because of the law of physics. It takes a certain amount of energy to move a specific mass over a prescribed distance regardless of the form of locomotion. (It takes more energy to swim a mile than walk a mile, however, because now you are moving a mass through water.)

"The overwhelming advantage of walking," claims Dr. Cooper, "is that it can be done by anyone, anytime, anyplace. It doesn't even look like exercise. For those who are timid about being conspicuous, this can be a deciding difference."

Cons: The long-distance runner, after getting over his ire at not burning any more energy running a mile in five minutes than someone who walks it in 20, suddenly realizes that he is four times more efficient in his fitness regimen. Or put it another way, walking is less efficient.

"It takes a greater period of time to accomplish the same energy expenditure," explains David L. Costill. And Dr. Cooper agrees: "It consumes more time per session."

This is practically the only negative comment that can be made about walking as a fitness activity.

Aerobics points per hour	3 (3 m.p.h.)
Calories burned per hour	210 (3 m.p.h.)
Mets	3-4 (3 m.p.h.)
Interest level	good
Injury risk level	almost none
Rating	* * *

6. STATIONARY RUNNING

Pros: This is one of the few sports you can engage in and watch television at the same time (which, come to think of it, may not be an advantage). Stationary running differs from ordinary running only in that you do not go anywhere. As a result, you can do it in any room in your house, or sometimes add some extra movement and run through your house. Sometimes I will be lying in bed reading a book before going to sleep, and my wife will come jogging past, dressed in her underwear, going "hup-hup-hup," sometimes making faces at me.

Stationary running is not as efficient as actual running in terms of either fat metabolized or calories burned, but it is still much more efficient than most other activities. For instance, Dr. Cooper allows you to score twice as many Aerobics points for stationary running as he does for handball, squash or basketball. He claims it has all the advantages of regular running except time, then adds, "Even if you've chosen running, swimming or cycling as your basic exercise, running in place can easily be substituted on those rainy or cold days when you can't get outdoors, or those busy days when you can't get to the swimming pool." The embarrassment factor also is zero.

Cons: Boredom. For those people who find running unstimulating, a variation of that exercise where you lose the advantage of changing scenery is doubly unstimulating. As a result, most people who do stationary running, probably do less of it than someone who goes to the extra trouble to run outdoors or in a gym. The risk of injury, particularly to the arches, might be somewhat higher, since more up-and-down pounding is involved. But since stationary runners probably exercise for shorter periods of time, they would be less likely to reach the danger threshold.

Aerobics points per hour	24 (80-90 steps per minute)
Calories burned per hour	400*
Interest level	low
Injury risk level	low
Rating	* * *

7. STATIONARY CYCLING

Stationary cycling, using an exercise bicycle in your home, is to regular cycling as stationary running is to regular running. The pros and cons—convenience vs. boredom—apply too, the only major difference being that it costs $125 for a good exercise cycle. (A rack stand which permits you to utilize your regular bike costs around $12.) Most good exercise cycles come equipped with a tension lever which permits you to increase your difficulty in pedaling, as well as a speedometer that gives you an indication as to how fast you might be traveling outdoors. One major advantage stationary cycling has over its outdoor variety is you never have to worry about colliding with a car.

Aerobics points per hour	20 (20 m.p.h.)
Calories burned per hour	660 (13 m.p.h.)
Mets	8-9 (13 m.p.h.)
Interest level	low
Injury risk level	none
Rating	* * *

8. RACQUETBALL

Pros: Here is another exercise (in addition to cross-country skiing) that Dr. Kenneth Cooper overlooked when he wrote *Aerobics* in 1968. He still failed to discover racquetball by *The New Aerobics* in 1970. (Small wonder: there was not one single racquetball club in the United States in that year.) *Aerobics for Women* (1972) also ignores the sport, although promoters of racquetball insist that it is a type of activity that women can learn with ease. However, when Dr. Cooper constructed his Aerobics Center in Dallas, he included two racquetball courts and says he now considers it one of the best fitness activities of its kind.

---

* Estimated.

Racquetball proponents cite its main advantage as being "fun." Chuck Sheftel, instructor at the Mid-Town Court House in Chicago insists, "The main assets of racquetball are that it is easy to learn, and there is great motion. Your body just flies. You dive. You glide. You slide on the courts, and I like that feeling."

Racquetball's ease in learning comes from its being played with short, light instruments (the racquets) which are easily handled. A person with moderate coordination can learn to hit the ball, and since the sport is played against four walls in a restricted space, the ball always bounces back—unlike tennis where it may bounce into the woods. The rules are relatively simple: if you are serving and your opponent misses, you score a point.

Perhaps one of the greatest appeals of racquetball, however, is that it is a game of finesse and strategy. A player who controls center court controls his opponent. Balls bouncing off the walls, front back and side, at odd angles provide a variety of situations during games.

Also, racquetball is played in clubs where a social atmosphere prevails. The basic equipment for the sport is inexpensive: $24 for a racquet, $1.00-$1.50 for a ball good for 40-50 games. It is a very efficient form of exercise for weight loss: 600 calories per hour for the average player, with professionals supposedly burning energy at the rate of 1000 calories per hour.

Cons: Although a social atmosphere prevails, racquetball today is mostly a young persons' sport. This eventually will change as those in their 20s and 30s continue playing into their 30s and 40s—and beyond. Although the basic equipment is inexpensive, court time is not: $9-$12 an hour in most clubs.

As for Aerobics points, Dr. Cooper rates an hour of handball, squash and basketball as worth approximately eight points. Racquetball would fall in this same category, perhaps slightly higher. This is for continuous activity and does not include breaks. However, a proficient player, who knows how to hold center court and plays an opponent of lesser ability, can run him all over the court, up to the front wall, back to the rear wall, without taking more than one or two steps to hit the ball. Racquetball, like tennis, is best played between players of equal ability—which raises the problem of finding a partner before being able to play. Because of the sport's popularity, obtaining court time (particularly immediately after work and on weekends) is no easy task.

And because racquetball is a game of quick sprints—a burst here, a burst there—David Costill feels it and other similar sports are of lesser benefit than sports such as swimming, running or cycling where energy is long and sustained.

"You don't turn on the fat metabolism as much by a little burst here and a little burst there," he suggests. "There is probably some sustained activity that turns on these mechanisms but not as fully as you would with low-level exercise. With high-intensity work, you burn up sugars as your source of energy. That's great as far as developing musculature, but it doesn't do much for fat metabolism."

As a result, one danger in racquetball is that, because players work up such a good sweat playing the game, they may consider themselves in better cardiovascular shape than actually is the case. The sudden starts and stops of the sport also provide much greater stress than in the so-called "low-level" activities such as running, swimming and jogging.

Because it is easy to learn and because it is a weekend sport, players often come to the courts in relatively poor physical condition. I noticed a number of grossly overweight individuals in my visits to racquetball courts. Nobody would consider racing a mile or a marathon without steady, continuous preparation. But overweight, undertrained weekend athletes often show up at racquetball courts, having paid for an hour's court time and determined to make full use of it in a sport that will place more sudden stress on their body than running a mile or a marathon.

The threat of heart attack, thus, is real and undoubtedly will increase as those in their 20s and their 30s continue playing into their 40s and 50s.

This possibly overstates the dangers, but people interested in participating in this growing and exciting sport probably should train for it (by running, swimming, cycling or variations of other four-star activities). The risk of injury in racquetball is relatively high, from pulled muscles to twisted ankles to collisions with the wall (or opponents) or being hit in the eye with a ball—but that should not discourage anyone from playing the sport as long as they take proper precautions.

Aerobics points per hour	8
Calories burned per hour	600
Mets	8-9
Interest level	very high
Injury risk level	high
Rating	* * *

9. HANDBALL

Pros: Handball players are presently suffering hard times, because they are having a difficult time preserving their court time against the onslought of racquetball players. When I visited the Lake Shore Athletic Club in Chicago recently to sample the sport, I noticed a sign in the locker room stating that the previously sacrosanct hours between 5 and 7 p.m. each weekday, where once only handballers could take court, were now being opened up to racquetball players. It is the first crumbling of the wall for many of these all-male athletic clubs, like first letting women to eat in the dining rooms. On the other hand, the construction of new racquetball courts (which also permit handball playing) opens new vistas for the game. (Squash, played on slightly different courts using longer handled racquets, seems, at least temporarily, out of vogue.)

Dr. Cooper points out that handball, along with basketball and squash, has "the immediate advantage of competition." (This could be considered a disadvantage as well). He points out that the astronauts, a highly competitive group, liked the sport. The risk of injury is probably less for handball players than racquetball players for the simple reason that you won't get hit in the face with a racquet.

Handball is unquestionably a superior sport to racquetball in the physical demands it places on a player. It requires more upper-body strength and agility, because the player hits the ball with a gloved hand instead of a light racquet. (Your hands will hurt unless they are conditioned to the ball's impact.) Since a player uses both hands, it helps to be somewhat ambidextrous.

One difference between the sports is that the ball doesn't fly off the wall, or racquet, at you quite as quickly in handball as in racquetball. Speed is less essential. This seems to be an advantage for older competitors, and Masters competition in handball began long before Masters competition in track and field or swimming. In fact, David Pain, founder of the Masters track movement, got his inspiration from having originally been a handball player.

There also is a camaraderie and sense of pride (that they are playing a *tougher* sport) that you sense among handball players as opposed to racquetball players. (You see somewhat the same distinction between marathon runners and joggers, although with less antagonism between the two groups; joggers aren't stealing the marathon player's courts.) Handballers often are fanatic in their belief that they have discovered the true sport. It becomes a religion for them (as it does with marathoners, too).

Cons: Basically, the same as with racquetball, with the addition being that handball is a much more difficult sport to learn the first time you visit the court. (It is much more difficult to hit a ball properly with a cupped hand, especially your left one if you are right-handed, than with a racquet.) For this reason, handball is a sport that people pick up while they are still in their 20s or not at all. Once having picked it up, however, they are likely to still be playing it into their 60s. Although the astronauts enjoyed the sport, one of them also had a non-fatal heart attack while playing it.

Handball players probably move around the court less than racquetball players, thus are even less likely to trigger their fat-burning metabolism. For this reason, plus the difficulty in acquiring the necessary skills to play it well, handball ranks lower as a fitness activity. If you love the sport, however, this should not discourage you.

Aerobics points per hour	8
Calories burned per hour	600
Mets	8-9
Interest level	high
Injury risk level	medium
Rating	* *

10. BASKETBALL

Pros: Probably no other sport, with the possible exception of the decathlon (which in one sense is 10 sports), better blends all the athletic disciplines into one.

Tom Heinsohn, coach of the Boston Celtics, says, "Basketball is a game that is a combination of ballet and wrestling."

To succeed in basketball, you not only need agility, intelligence and strength, but you also need the endurance of a long-distance runner.

Dr. Cooper states that an hour of continuous basketball results in nine Aerobics points. I feel he is being conservative. Perhaps he merely is thinking of basketball played similar to that in the "slow-break" league in Michigan City, where rules require the offensive team to walk the ball into the forecourt. In that case, I would agree with him. But in the running game that until a few years ago I played with friends in our church gymnasium, I suspect the point totals could go higher. A runner who covers 10 miles in an hour scores 60 points, and I would suspect that a basketball player playing at a comparable level of ability would earn double the points Dr. Cooper allows. Basketball, played at a peak of intensity, requires almost continuous running—even if it is start and stop.

For some reason, Dr. Johnson's energy expenditure charts fail to include basketball. Another calorie chart rates half-court basketball at 286 calories, or less than cycling six m.p.h. That would have to be a rather tepid game. The number of calories burned per hour should at least equal those burned in handball, or 600 calories. Diet physiologist Marcus Sorenson says he enjoys playing one-on-one basketball when he can find a player of equal ability and says he once lost 25 pounds in seven days in this way.

Cons: Unfortunately, basketball is a sport that places a premium on height. Most Americans much shorter than six feet get weeded out of their high school basketball programs at an early age, thus rarely develop the skills they might learn if they played the sport regularly.

Because basketball is a contact sport (if you don't think so, watch any NBA game), the risk of injury is extremely high. Very few basketball players continue their sport much beyond their 20s—or even *into* their 20s. Added to that is the problem that to be played properly you need 10 players, a gymnasium and (preferably) a referee. Even Marc Sorenson admits difficulty finding one-on-one opponents.

Thus, despite its high potential for fitness, basketball ranks low as an exercise simply because too few people will play it or play it properly. Shooting baskets in your back yard isn't basketball; it's shooting baskets.

Aerobics points per hour	9
Calories burned per hour	286
Mets	7-8
Interest level	high
Injury risk level	high
Rating	* *

11. TENNIS

Pros: Tennis is a very graceful game. It is a game requiring skill and agility. It is also a game which ranks well in terms of caloric expenditure, since an hour of tennis burns 420 calories. Dr. Cooper suggests that one set of singles, about 20 minutes of play, will earn 1.5 points, thus 4.5 points per hour. Tennis uses 6-7 mets.

Although tennis once was considered a rich man's sport and a game for sissies, it has shed much of that image within the last decade—at least in the public press. I suspect it is partly because we are getting an increasing number of tennis players on the sports staffs of our daily newspapers. When managing editors started demanding journalism degrees for new staffers, they unconsciously changed the tone of their sports pages.

Cons: Probably the largest negative factor of tennis is testament to its popularity. Try to find an unoccupied court in any well-populated area on the weekend or in the evenings. Equipment for tennis, if you are not too fashion-conscious, is only moderately expensive ($15 and up for a racquet). But if you want to play , court time is $12-16 an hour.

Sometimes, during the summer when I am searching for a tennis court, I get on my bicycle and pedal from one court to another, often spending nearly an hour in my search and covering a half-dozen or more miles. This normally would do wonders for a person's cardiovascular fitness, but I don't need it, and I suspect the majority of tennis players in search of a court do so in their 280-Z's.

Probably the most negative comment that can be made about tennis is that the people who play it think they are staying fit when they are not. Tennis does wonders for your spirit but very little for your cardiovascular system. Most tennis players could achieve better fitness if they did leave their 280-Z's at home and rode bicycles to the courts, or still better used one or more of the four-star activities to get in shape off-season and on days when they were not playing.

I commented thusly in a letter to Shepherd Campbell, editor of *Tennis,* and afterwards feared that I might have offended him. Not so. He wrote back, "Your description of tennis conditions is a virtual paraphrase of a maxim we quote around here all the time; namely, that you should get in shape to play tennis and not play tennis to get in shape."

One more negative comment: A cigarette company is allowed to sponsor the women's professional tennis tour. I know of at least one physician who resigned from the United States Lawn Tennis Association in protest for this reason. His name is Frank L. Rosen, M.D., of Maplewood, N.J., and I am mailing him an autographed copy of this book as a show of support. When I went to see Chris Evert play Margaret Court this winter, I almost suffered nicotine poisoning sitting in the gallery.

Aerobics points per hour	4.5
Calories burned per hour	420
Mets	6-7
Interest level	high
Injury risk level	low
Rating	**

12. DOWNHILL SKIING

Pros: The pros and cons that apply to tennis do so also for downhill skiing, a sport that is both difficult to learn and beautiful when you learn it. Dr. Cooper suggests that downhill skiing earns the participant six Aerobics points for an hour, counting time actively skiing. This may cause a problem in calibrating points, since a skier might spend an entire weekend at a ski resort and spend less than an hour actually skiing. Much more time would be consumed waiting in lift lines or standing poised at the top of the hill, gaining courage to go downhill (or standing poised at the bar talking about it afterwards).

A skier who knows his art, however, will probably earn at least that many points, because he will make more runs and more active runs. He also will gain some credit for the cross-country skiing he does between runs. In fact, he may achieve *most* of his cardiovascular fitness this way. Dr. Johnson fails to establish an energy expenditure value for downhill skiing. (Cross-country skiing burns 600 calories per hour at 10 m.p.h., and water skiing burns 480 calories.) An educated guess at the calorie consumption for downhill skiers (including standing-around time) would be 350 calories, or the same as for horseback riding and square dancing.

Cons: Skiing is probably the most expensive sport you can indulge in aside from automobile racing (for which you earn no Aerobics points). Those actively involved in the sport, who own the best equipment and travel to the best resorts, find themselves with a four-figure habit, financially speaking.

Skiing shares another element with auto racing: danger. It is a rare skier, no matter how gifted, who has not suffered, at one time or another, a serious, incapacitating injury, usually a broken bone.

Back in the 1950s, when I was engaged to be married, I belonged to a ski club in Chicago. My future wife was horrified, on attending our club's annual meeting, to learn about several memorial awards for members killed on ski trips. These deaths occurred not on the slopes but in car accidents driving home from the slopes. Typically, skiers in the Midwest work at their regular jobs on Friday, drive half the night to reach northern resorts, ski all day Saturday, party late Saturday night, ski all day Sunday and drive half the night to get home. They form a high-accident-risk group, both late on the slopes Sunday as well as driving home.

In fact, I suspect a lot of benefits of the weekend of exercise get washed away during the parties Saturday nights. Skiing remains a graceful sport, like tennis, but most fitness benefits come from efforts its participants make to get in shape to do it.

Aerobics points per hour	6
Calories burned per hour	350*
Mets	6-7
Interest level	exceptionally high
Injury risk level	exceptionally high
Rating	*

* Estimated.

13. GOLF

Pros: The best comment that need be said about golf is that it can be a very enjoyable activity—as long as your putts are dropping. I used to fool around with golf on a fairly regular basis when I was younger and had a low score of 89. Now that I have salved my ego, I must admit that, during the once-or-so-a-year occasion I now play, I am lucky to get under 120. Very lucky.

Dr. Cooper rates golf as worth 1.5 points per nine holes. If you pull your bag on a cart, golf takes 3-4 mets, or the same as horseshoe pitching. If you climb in an electric cart, the met level sinks to 2-3, or the same as typing and bartending.

Cons: One of my good friends, Jim O'Neil of Sacramento, Calif., now runs marathons and has won national championships and set Masters records in the 50s age division, but he once was a moderately low-handicap golfer. He has a lifetime best of 80. On Nov. 3, 1972, he set a world record of sorts by playing 18 holes of golf in 47:17, running between strokes. His score during this combination golf/sprint was 99. Later, Jim Fries of Fresno bettered O'Neil's record with 38:12 and a score of 81. A golfer from Nebraska reportedly did 18 in 30:10.

O'Neil, Fries and the Nebraska golfer probably are among the few individuals to ever attain much physical fitness from the sport which Dr. Paul Dudley White once said was "a good way to spoil a walk." Dr. Cooper's Aerobics tables seem to bear him out, since nine holes of golf (which would take approximately two hours to play) earn the participant 1.5 points. Two hours of moderately fast walking (six miles) earns the participant three points.

An hour of golf on Dr. Johnson's energy expenditure chart is worth 250 points, slightly less than the 255 points you earn at the rate of walking three miles an hour.

And golf is expensive.

(One further note about Jim O'Neil. He frequently trained for his long-distance races near, or on, the same country club course where he played golf in the afternoon. One time, a caddy at that club, whose income depended on people walking and using his services, commented to a friend of Jim's, "I don't understand that guy O'Neil. Every morning, I see him running up and down the street, but when he plays golf he takes a cart.")

Aerobics points per hour	0.75
Calories burned per hour	250
Mets	3-4 (walking)
	2-3 (riding)
Interest level	high
Injury risk level	non-existent
Rating	*

14. VARIOUS "PROFESSIONAL" SPORTS

Baseball, football, boxing and ice hockey share many of the same pros and cons as basketball. They are sports played by youngsters who rarely continue in those sports past their teens unless they are good enough (or big enough) to attract athletic scholarships or professional contracts. Invariably, those who do the later retire after the money runs out. Unless they take up another sport, they often become the most unfit, poorly conditioned individuals on their blocks. (One exception is Chuck Davey, who once fought for the world welterweight title against Kid Gavilan. At age 50, he now runs marathons.)

There are some areas where competition in these sports continues. In the area around St. Petersburg, Fla., there exist baseball leagues for men in their 60s and 70s. There is an ice hockey league in New York City for men over 35 that I know of only because Joseph Breu, who works in public relations for the American Medical Association, told me he sometimes plays in their games when he visits that city. He says he enjoys playing ice hockey with people his own age, because they have reactions similar to his. He no longer remains competitive with younger players. Competition in boxing and football for older athletes virtually is non-existent.

Variations on professional sports such as touch football and softball have pockets of popularity, but they provide very little in the way of cardiovascular fitness. Most professional sports, thus, can be rated together:

Aerobics points per hour:

Football	6
Hockey	9
Baseball	2*
Boxing	9*

* Estimated.

Calories burned per hour:
- Hockey — 400
- Boxing — 400*
- Football — 360*
- Baseball — 270*

Mets
- Boxing — 8-9*
- Hockey — 7-8
- Touch Football — 7-8
- Baseball — 4-5*
- Interest level — high
- Injury risk level — extremely high
- Rating — *

15. CALISTHENICS AND WEIGHT LIFTING

Pros: When he first wrote *Aerobics*, Dr. Cooper stated that calisthenics, as well as weight lifting and isometrics, often increased body strength but did little to improve cardiovascular fitness. They did not even make his list of recommended exercises, "despite the fact that most exercise books are *based* on one of these three, especially calisthenics."

Dr. Johnson also failed to include calisthenics on his energy expenditure list, although he rated gardening as burning 220 calories and rowing at 300. (Calisthenics are listed on the mets table at the 4-5 level, along with raking leaves and paper hanging.)

Nevertheless, calisthenics can form an important part of an individual's total fitness program—but only a part. Calisthenics are best used as a warming-up exercise before performing one of the higher ranked sports. The same is true for weight lifting, which could be a good supplemental exercise for some of the activities, such as cycling or jogging, which do relatively little for the upper body.

Cons: There are few hazards in a calisthenic-type regimen, but there is a subtle danger in weight lifting, particularly when practiced at the high levels of competition. The sport makes almost no aerobic demands on the body, and most weight lifters try to "bulk-up," by going on high protein diets, with the resulting risk of high cholesterol. When they cease lifting, their weight may eventually become fat unless they engage in some other exercise program. If weight lifting is done properly, there is probably little danger of becoming "muscle-bound," but weight lifting probably should be used in combination with stretching exercises to maintain flexibility.

Aerobic points per hour	minimal
Calories burned per hour	300*
Mets	4-5
Interest level	very low
Injury risk level	low
Rating	*

16. ISOMETRICS

Pros: Exercising through isometrics no longer is at the fad level it was during the mid-1960s, when isometrics was hailed as the miracle exercise by everyone from professional football teams to overweight housewives. "How to Move Inches Without Moving an Inch," was the article in one magazine.

Isometrics was a counterpart to isotonics, which was the label for exercises involving movement (pull-ups, push-ups, etc.). In isometrics, you flex the muscle without moving it.

In terms of energy expenditure, I would guess 160 calories might be a good figure, halfway between the 140 you burn by simply standing still and the 180 burned in domestic work. Isometrics fails to make the mets list.

At the height of the isometrics fad, I wrote an article for *Today's Heath* (published by the American Medical Association) entitled "Let's Tell the Truth About Isometrics." It was a debunking article, as the title would indicate. My conclusion was that there was a limited need for isometrics. One need was therapeutic for people with limbs immobilized in casts who could not exercise them isotonically. Another use was in strength tests, to measure the effect of isotonics. Isometrics also had advantages in shaping parts of the body such as flabby stomach muscles. I admitted that isometrics had some value as a supplemental exercise in a training regimen that also included isotonic exercises such as running and walking, but I was definitely negative.

So what did *Today's Health* do but include with this article

---

* Estimated.

diagrams and descriptions of how to do a half-dozen isometric exercises! I do not intend to include them here.

Cons: According to Dr. Cooper, "Isometric exercises are capable of increasing the size and strength of individual skeletal muscles, but they have no significant effect on overall health, especially on the pulmonary and cardiovascular systems. There is no increase in oxygen consumption and consequently minimal, if any, training effect."

Probably the most negative thing that can be said about isometrics is that anyone who did them thinking he was helping himself become physically fit was kidding himself.

Aerobics points per hour	none
Calories burned per hour	160
Mets	no rating
Interest level	very low
Injury risk level	moderately low
Rating	no stars

And at the risk of stating the obvious, there also are no benefits, in terms of either cardiovascular fitness or in terms of energy expenditure, as pleasureful as they may make you feel, either by taking a sauna bath or lounging in a Jacuzzi.

And no health benefits can be earned *writing* about sports. I think I'll go out for a run.

15
The Semi-Obligatory Physical Examination Disclaimer

We are nearing that magic part of any exercise book when, having heaped upon you the best in medical advice, convinced you that you need to improve your physical fitness and having given you suggestions as to the best means of achieving that end, we are goint to push you out the door clad in Sears' best sweatsuit with a pair of Adidas flats on your feet.

But before that moment, a brief message. It is time for the semi-obligatory disclaimer which appears in virtually every article and/or book written about physical fitness. Namely: *you should not endulge in any strenuous athletic activity without first obtaining a thorough physical examination from a doctor.*

Presumably, this inoculates the author against recourse from the widows of husbands who have charged out of the house bent on extending their lifespan, only to die on the doorstep from a heart attack. "He should have had that physical," the author can claim, salving his conscience.

I have written the semi-obligatory physical examination disclaimer, in many variations, dozens of times in connection with health articles. You probably already have tripped over it several times in this book. But I confess I am skeptical about the thoroughness of the average physical examination. Others also have expressed skepticism, including Richard Spark, M.D., an associate clinical professor at Harvard Medical School who wrote an article in the *New York Times Magazine*, July 25, 1976, entitled, "The Case Against Regular Physicals." Dr. Spark's point was that they found too little and cost too much. Kenneth H. Cooper, M.D., disagrees with this point of view. He considers a stress test absolutely necessary before starting to exercise, and also believes every man over 40 should have an annual sigmoidoscopy exam (of the rectum and lower bowel) to protect against cancer. 101,000 Americans contract rectal cancer each year, and 51,000 of them die from it. So who do we believe?

We are all creatures of our own experiences, and back in high school I appeared at our family physician's office one afternoon for an annual examination. He listened to my heart, which apparently was beating too strongly. (One reason was that instead of taking a bus, I had walked three miles from school to his office then run up the stairs, but I failed to tell him that.) It was early fall and I was having my usual hay fever problems, which he overdiagnosed as asthma. The doctor recommended I not engage in physical activity for a year. This meant I could not compete in cross-country or track my junior year in high school, but having just transferred schools I was ineligible, anyway.

So I obeyed and one year later reported to that physician again. He told me to avoid physical activity *forever!* I might damage my heart. That information disturbed me. But doctor knows best, and I abandoned cross-country again that fall. Later, I decided to ignore what the doctor told me and went out for track the spring of my senior year, badly conditioned and a bit fearful. I survived and have been in near-continuous physical activity since, a time period that spans four decades.

This is one reason why I distrust the average doctor's views on physical fitness. One stole from me my high school athletic career. Please notice I said *average* doctor. I would not rate someone such as Ken Cooper, or George Sheehan, or Noel Nequin, or anyone else who actively engages in physical activity as average doctors. They would not have made that early doctor's mistake. For it was a mistake, a bad diagnosis, a case of malpractice, since obeying him might have affected my health negatively. Several decades later, x-rays of my heart are shown at medical meetings as an example of what a healthy heart looks like.

While I was at Runner's Mecca, I talked with Rory Donaldson, an executive with the National Jogging Association and editor of that organization's publication, *The Jogger*. Rory refuses to be seen by a physician who is not a fellow runner. In fact, he even said he spent a half-year looking all over Washington, D.C., to find a *dentist* who also ran. I thought his position extreme, but he told me, "I don't want anybody involved with my health, even a dentist, normalizing me against the rest of the population." (My dentist in Long Beach, Tom Talaga, does not jog, but he goes cross-country skiing. We also sometimes play basketball together.)

Rory was right. The problem is that the average doctor, in his regular practice, sees only average people. More than likely, he sees only those among the average people who, often through lack of physical activity, have allowed their health to deteriorate to the point where they now need above-average treatment. What they actually needed was preventive medicine before they reported to their doctor's office. So the average doctor does not know how to react to the above-average individual: a person who either is an athlete or who has the desire (after reading this book) to become an athlete.

Fortunately, this is changing. More and more physicians are becoming involved in physical fitness programs of their own. The American Medical Joggers Association, for example, has a membership of more than 1000, and many of them do not merely jog but compete often in full-distance marathons. Recently, while visiting Galveston, Tex., I went for a run along the seawall early one morning and fell in with a young runner putting in a 10-mile workout before attending classes at the University of Texas Medical Branch, where he was studying to become a physician. Until recently, medical students never had the time nor *took* the time to remain active physically. This is changing.

The previous spring, I was asked by the father of a local high school runner for advice. His son John Bradley, a 4:36 miler on the track team and a friend of my son, suffered chest pains on several occasions that caused him to drop out of several races. I doubted there were any cardiac problems in someone apparently so healthy, but it seemed prudent to be overcautious. A stress test was advised. To assure the father, I said I would go to the hospital and watch the test administered.

Having had numerous tests myself, I assumed the hospital would have, at minimum, an inexpensive treadmill on which subjects could walk or possibly jog at a slow pace while being monitored by an electrocardiogram machine. But ours is a small town, and when I arrived at the testing room I realized they still used the standard step box for stress tests. You go up one side—one, two—then down the other, turn around and keep repeating the process. Several minutes of such activity supposedly raises your heart beat so a trained observer can detect abnormalities on the ECG.*

I was skeptical, but on the other hand cardiologist George Sheehan, M.D., once told me he can learn as much from a simple step test as he can from one on a treadmill. Of course, as I said earlier, George Sheehan is not an average doctor. In addition to having run the Boston Marathon 15 successive years, he writes a monthly medical column for *Runner's World*. The person testing the young miler was not George Sheehan. She was a nurse, and while many nurses, particularly the new breed of nurse practitioners, are more competent in performing certain duties than physicians, it became soon apparent that she did not know how to adequately test a well-conditioned athlete.

The young miler started going up and down the step. The nurse attempted to slow him down, fearing he was going too fast. After several minutes of bouncing over the steps, the miler plunged onto an examining table, and the nurse began attaching electrodes to his chest. I had a hard time suppressing a smile, because I anticipated what would happen. Sure enough, by the time she got the ECG machine rolling, his heart had slowed to normal.

The nurse sighed and asked him to repeat the test—this time faster—and she raced to get the ECG attached before his heart slowed, apparently without much more luck. Eventually, the

---

* While I was writing this chapter there was an item in our local newspaper that one of the other two hospitals in town had just installed an expensive treadmill and console similar to the one used by Dr. Hellerstein and Barry Franklin in Cleveland.

physician, a general practitioner, stepped into the room, examined the ECG printouts and decided the miler probably was fit. He returned to running and was good enough to place 26th in the state cross-country meet the following fall. But I wonder if 20 years from now John Bradley will look back on that physical examination with the same skepticism that I recall from my youthful medical confrontation. Probably not, because physicians are becoming increasingly involved in sports medicine.

I used to get physical examinations from that same physician (whom I still call occasionally when I need the prescription for my dandruff shampoo refilled), but he buzzed in and out so rapidly I doubted the thoroughness of his findings. It was mostly a lack of communication. More recently, I have had physical examinations done by exercise physiologists such as David L. Costill at the Human Performance Laboratory at Ball State University, or by Michael L. Pollock at Ken Cooper's Institute for Aerobics Research in Dallas. I never wind up paying for these exams, because physiologists usually are looking for an excuse to study me. In fact, sometimes, they do the paying.

The test Mike Pollock gave me in November 1976 is perhaps typical of the examinations you receive at such performance laboratories. When I talked to Mike by telephone the day before, he asked me to refrain from eating any food or drinking anything other than water for 12 hours before the test. I flew into Dallas early in the morning and reported to the Institute, in a half-basement about a half-mile down the street from the Aerobics Center where Dr. Cooper practices.

Soon after my arrival, they took blood samples from my arm, something competitive runners must get used to since physiologists constantly are bleeding us. Laboratory tests indicated my levels as: cholesterol, 181 (very low); triglycerides, 44 (extremely low); glucose, 100 (low), and uric acid, 5.6 (very low). My resting blood pressure showed a systolic reading of 110 and a diastolic pressure of 68. My resting pulse rate was 32 beats per minute seated. (Lying down, I clocked 29.) My pride in that accomplishment was tempered by the knowledge that an individual's pulse rate decreases with age at the rate of about one beat per year. (Presumably, if we accept that standard, once I reach the age of 77 my pulse rate will be down to one thundering beat per minute. The following year: good-bye.)

Pollock also measured my body fat, and while in previous examinations physiologists used calipers to determine the thickness of my skin in nearly a dozen areas, he used a more precise method: he tried to drown me. I sat strapped onto a scale in a large tank of water, and when he directed I submerged my head. He later informed me I had 7.1% body fat. At the time of the test, I was somewhat heavier than the 135 pounds at which I have had some of my best racing performances but not quite as heavy as the 145 I weigh while writing this chapter. My weight varies depending on my level of training (if I fail to modify my diet, I gain weight just as rapidly as other people) and depending on the time of year (since I usually weigh myself after a workout, summer weights are lower because of water lost during excessive persperation).

That completed, I moved to another room, at the center of which was a treadmill—actually a belt that could be activated to move as fast as 20 m.p.h. to simulate an all-out sprint or tilted to simulate running up a hill. There were rails in front and to the side of the treadmill to assist the runner in getting on and off the moving belt, and to prevent him from launching himself into space. Beside the belt were various measuring machines, including an electrocardiograph and a mask attached to a tube for collecting breath samples. It was similar to the model on which I had run on numerous occasions at the Human Performance Laboratory at Ball State University under the supervision of David L. Costill.

After a brief warmup run of several minutes, electrocardiograph leads were attached to my chest. My resting pulse rate, measured earlier at 32, was up to 38 standing on the treadmill. I placed the mouthpiece from the collection device into my mouth; a clip went over my nose. All my breathing would be done through this breathing apparatus, which would permit measurment of my maximum oxygen uptake. No attempt was made to monitor my temperature, although in previous tests at Ball State I had run with a rectal thermometer in place during three two-hour sessions, three days in succession, to measure the effects of liquids (including Gatorade) in controlling body temperature. At the end of each two-hour session, Dave Costill stuck a tube through my nose and pumped my stomach to see how much liquid remained unabsorbed. On another occasion, I had my thigh biopsied: a piece of tissue sliced out of it to determine my ratio of fast-twitch vs. slow-twitch fibers. (I am 61% slow twitch, which presumably is one reason I am effective at running long-distances.) All this for science.

The treadmill started moving and, grasping the side-rails, I jumped onto it, holding on until my pace equaled that of the moving belt. Then I released my grip and continued to run as I would on an outdoor track. I remembered the words of the queen in Alice in Wonderland: "You have to run fast just to stay where you are."

The belt was moving at 9.5 miles per hour, slightly slower than a six-minute pace per mile. At one minute, my pulse rate reached 117 beats per minute, but by two it dropped to 112 as I became accustomed to the peculiar rhythm necessary for running on the treadmill and became more efficient in my movements. Running a steady treadmill pace takes a certain peculiar skill, similar in some respects to running high hurdles. You have to run straight, the way a hurdler runs in his lane. You must run smoothly. You need to maintain concentration, because if you unconsciously slow down you find yourself losing ground and threatened with a painful fall.

One of the most frequently asked question to a marathon runner is, "What do you think about while you're running all that time?" What you think about, if you're maximizing your potential, is putting one foot in front of another, then putting the next foot in front of it. It takes maximum concentration to succeed in any sport, and long-distance running is no exception. After talking to many race drivers, I am convinced concentration, even more than quick reflexes, is the single skill or ability that permits some individuals to succeed in races like the Indianapolis 500 while others fail. Quite frequently, when a runner begins dropping off the pace in a long-distance race, it is not his legs that go but rather his concentration. When I was running for two-hour periods on Dave Costill's treadmill, I refused to permit anyone to stand directly in front of me, because it interfered with my concentration. Dave usually stood off to the side when he talked to me.

After three minutes, the treadmill grade was raised to 2.5% to increase the stress. Otherwise, I might be running all morning before reaching the point where I could go no farther, the point at which they measure my maximum oxygen uptake. My pulse rate at three minutes was 118. At four, it was 129. At five, they raised the grade to 5%, and my pulse moved steadily up into the 140s. It reached 151 when they raised the grade once more to 7.5% at seven minutes.

This is a fairly severe grade. On a highway with that grade, there probably would be a sign warning trucks to shift to second gear. Only the steepest roads go much higher. During the telecast of the 1976 Olympic Marathon, one of the broadcasters described a hill on the course as having a 33% grade, which was absurd. The high-banked turns at the Daytona Motor Speedway are 31 degrees. I have been on them, and you can barely stand, much less walk up them.

At 7 1/2 minutes, my pulse reached 155 beats. At each succeeding half-minute from then on, its steady progress upward was recorded: 155 again, 157, 158, 158 again, 159 at 10 minutes.

Every so often, Mike Pollock would ask how I felt. I had three signals by which I could reply. Thumbs up meant I felt fine. Thumbs sideways meant I was beginning to tire. Thumbs down meant to stop the treadmill. Coming up to 10 minutes, my breath was coming in gasps and I knew I was nearing the point of total fatigue. I gave the thumbs sideways signal. Past 10 minutes and it was thumbs down, and Mike shouted to hold on to the next 15-second break.

I tried to imagine myself coming down the final straightaway in the 1500-meter run. "Sprint!" I shouted at myself. "Sprint!" Two summers before in the 1500 at the National Masters Championships at White Plains, N.Y., I had come onto the backstretch in the final lap in seventh place, well behind the leader Albie Thomas of Australia. With a closing surge, I passed everyone ahead of me except Thomas, running 4:06.1. (According to Ken Young's figures, that was the equivalent of approximately 3:40 by a younger runner.) I tried to recapture that moment there on the treadmill but failed. Perhaps physiologists should mount a television screen before their treadmills with videotapes of the backs of other runners.

When I stopped at 10:15, my pulse rate had reached a maximum of 160 beats. I was soaked with sweat, tired but not exhausted. I worried that I had not pushed myself to my maximum. I recovered rapidly. At the end of one minute, my pulse reached 77 beats; my blood pressure, 210 over 90. By two minutes, my pulse dropped to 60, and it remained at that steady level through five minutes when my blood pressure lowered to 120 over 80.

Mike Pollock said I had one premature beat during recovery, but he considered it nothing to be concerned about. Yet that premature beat could be a hint of what might be my fate if I did not exercise so vigorously. I remembered again my father, dead of a heart attack at age 69. He was overweight and had only recently begun smoking cigarettes again after nearly 15 years of abstinence.

I do not consider myself immune from heart attack, nor do I run for immunity. I could be struck by an arrythmia as was the case with Jim Shettler. I could even embarrass myself and my publishers by having a myocardial infarction in the midst of a marathon, maybe becoming the one case that will disprove Tom Bassler's theories about immunity for marathon runners. The odds, however, are against it.

Mike Pollock later computed my maximum oxygen uptake at 69.38. This compared with a 70.8 reading in 1968 when I was 37 years old. In 1971, I had reached a value of 62.7. According to measurements made by J. L. Hodgson of the University of Minnesota, the expected maximum oxygen uptake for a 45-year-old man who was "moderately active" would have been 41.8. I expressed my sorrow that the test was not done when I was in peak physical condition, as in the summer of 1975. I thought I could push my uptake higher.

"Everybody always says that," commented Pollock, smiling. "But there probably would be little measurable difference."

The highest maximum oxygen uptake ever recorded by Mike Pollock was that of former University of Oregon distance runner, the late Steve Prefontaine, who once hit 84.4. At that point, *he* expressed the desire to come in sometime when he was really fit and push that record "out of sight."

One time, Dave Costill measured the maximum oxygen uptake of a trumpet player who came into the laboratory boasting of his vital capacity. "You need strong lungs to be able to hold high notes on the trumpet," he insisted. Costill measured him and found his value to be 24.8. He did not have the heart to tell the trumpet player that his capacity was "below average" and far beneath the marks that would be demonstrated by a competitive athlete.

After Mike Pollock compiled all of the records from the laboratory as well as from a psychological test given me, he was able to show me how I ranked on a coronary risk profile then being developed at the Institute for Aerobics Research. I scored zero points in personal history of heart attack, smoking habits, resting ECG and exercise ECG. I scored two points under family history of heart attack for a cross marked in the box, "Yes, over 50 years." I scored one point for "moderate tension." (As indicated previously, I suspect successful competitive runners fit more neatly into the Type A personality box than uncompetitive joggers.) I scored two points in the age factor category, merely for being between 40 and 49 years of age. My total coronary risk was five points, which rated me "low." To rate "very low," I would have to score between zero and four points.

Mike Pollock warned me, however, that this method of determining a person's coronary heart disease probability was still undergoing validation. "It may or may not prove effective as a predictive tool," he admitted.

What can we learn from such extensive testing programs? It often is difficult to assess the meaning of the statistics that spill out of the computers from physiologists such as Michael L. Pollock and David L. Costill. They tell me I am physically fit, but we all knew that before I mounted the treadmill. They show me the numbers, but often it is difficult for a layman to assess the meaning of such numbers. Often it is difficult even for a trained physiologist to determine the meaning of what he is collecting. On several occasions, I will point to one of the values on my chart and ask Dave or Mike what this means in terms of my ability to run a fast mile?

They smile softly and say, "Maybe in about 20 years, we will be able to tell you."

One study I am involved in will take at least that long to obtain definite results: an attempt by Costill to measure the physical deterioration of long-distance runners over their lifespan. Included in this study besides myself are Amby Burfoot, Ted Corbitt, Jim McDonagh and Lou Castagnola. Amby Burfoot won the Boston marathon in 1967 and has an alltime best of 2:14:28. Ted Corbitt ran the marathon in the 1952 Olympics and has run 100 miles in 13:33:06. Jim McDonagh made the Pan-American Games team in 1969 at age 45 and ran 2:28:49 the following year. Lou Castagnola had an all-time marathon best of 2:17:48 and once placed fourth at Boston.

The original measurements were made in 1968, and we were brought in again in 1971 for retesting. Although I have been measured several times since, Costill admits he is late in getting the others back in for follow-up. They will probably be retested this coming summer, too late for inclusion in this book.

By 1971, only one of those runners had retired from racing: Lou Castagnola. "We saw remarkable reversals in his fitness levels," Costill admitted. "He dropped back to the point where he looked like a typical middle-aged man. He still had good endurance, but his maximum oxygen uptake dropped from 78 down to about 47."

I asked Costill what he was learning from the numerous studies he and other physiologists were making on individuals exercising. "We are doing two things," he explained. "First, in order to convince people of the importance of physical activity, we can show them that, physiologically, there are benefits.

"Second, a lot of people ask: 'Will exercise make me live longer?' At this point, we can't say yes. But we are beginning to accumulate data in isolated specifics, studies of heart disease risk factors. We see certain changes that occur in fat levels of blood. The profiles normally associated with heart disease are markedly being altered by exercise. It's like saying that if you give up cigarettes you reduce your chances for lung cancer. The same is true with some of these factors. If you become more physically active, we have evidence that you reduce your risk of coronary disease. It's a matter of establishing a very difficult case, but I think in time the case will be very tight in that, definitely, your chances of living longer are better if you are physically active."

Dave Costill paused. "But unfortunately you never can do a control study, because individuals are individuals."

One recent study at the Human Performance Laboratory relates to diabetics, who have tremendous problems lowering their fat levels. "They not only cannot get sugar out of their blood," Costill said, "but they cannot get fats out, either. As a result, they develop heart disease 2-4 times faster than the normal individual who is not diabetic. That's why diabetics die fairly early of heart disease. We're working with them now, trying to show that an exercise program benefits diabetics because it helps remove sugar from the blood and remove demands for insulin. It also lowers certain types of blood fats."

David Costill summed up his case: "Exercise is good for the diabetic, but it also is good for the non-diabetic. We are convinced of that. I was never a salesman for exercise. I don't like to go around preaching it. But there is no question in my mind that there is a benefit to cardiovascular health."

In testing people of all ages, Dave Costill discovered few men in their 30s with heart problems. The curve showing the amount of deficiency, however, too a sharp turn upward in the 50-55 age group. In the 60 age group, he found that nearly everyone had some inadequacies with regard to oxygen supply for the heart muscle.

One of the problems with people past 40 who exercise is that many of them are athletes who laid off; many others are non-athletes who began jogging at age 35.

"The next thing that happens is that they run a few races and get competitive," Costill explained. "The danger is that they may have cardiovascular problems because of the aging degradations on the circulatory system. The greatest risk is those people who don't start activity until 35 or 40. For their own health and safety, they should be given a stress test."

Which brings us full-circle to the semi-obligatory physical examination disclaimer. Unfortunately, not everyone can afford to have as complete a physical examination as I normally obtain for free at either the Human Performance Laboratory or the Institute for Aerobics Research. Neither Costill nor Pollock is in the stress test business, although patients at the Cooper Clinic and members of the Aerobics Center receive tests for $85. Costill's laboratory charge $100.

If you receive a physical examination elsewhere, the average physician can examine a simple electrocardiograph taken while seated and evaluate it to determine if there are any obvious heart problems. Using a step test allows him to make a better observation. A somewhat more specialized cardiologist will test a person on a treadmill and obtain a still better picture of a person's capacity for exercise. But most physicians test persons to only 75% of their capacity for exercise, thus may miss abnormal readings that could appear if a person were tested to near 100%. And very few physicians know much about offering advice as to starting a training program. Finding the few physicians who do is an art in itself.

"If you are going to get a maximum stress test," admits Tom Bassler, M.D., "and you are an athlete in training, you will present the average doctor with a problem, because he won't be set up for you. He is set up for testing middle-aged executives. If you show up in your Adidas shoes and your track shorts, he won't know what to do. So you have to find a physician to whom other runners go, preferably a physician who runs the marathon."

Dr. Bassler suggests that one method of locating such a physician is by calling your local YMCA and asking to be directed to a cardiologist who knows something about running. That failing, the alternative, particularly for someone in a big city, is to begin calling nearby hospitals.

"You ask for the cardiology department," advises Dr. Bassler. "You talk to the nurse on duty, and ask her if there's someone on the staff who jogs. If she says no, you hang up and call another hospital, because if there is a doctor jogger usually everybody in the hospital knows it. Usually, it's some dumb nut doctor who nobody would ever refer anybody to. But that's the guy you want to give you your stress test."

So much for the semi-obligatory physical examination disclaimer. And remember, if you die of a heart attack during exercise or while jogging, be sure to have your widow call Tom Bassler.

16

Keeping It Up

According to the American Medical Association, *"There is one tried and true role for all those who are out of shape and want to start training: start slowly and increase the vigor and duration of the activity as your fitness improves. In time, you will be able to do with ease what was hard for you in the beginning."*

I'm borrowing that statement from the AMA, but with good reason: it is sound advice. Having competed as a runner for three decades, I should know everything there is to know about the sport, but I constantly am learning new tricks on how one gets in shape. I would like to pass some of them onto you.

For example, while writing this book I flew into San Diego one evening to spend some time with David H. R. Pain, founder of the Masters movement in track and a close, personal friend. David picked me up at the airport in his Toyota preparatory to having dinner at a nearby Chinese restaurant. Those following the so-called Marathon Life Style more often can be found eating in Chinese restaurants (where vegetables form an important part of most courses) or Italian restaurants (where pasta is equally important). After I climbed into his car, I glanced up and noticed a bumper sticker on the car parked in front of us, a Porsche. It read, "Distance Runners Keep It Up Longer."

It is a familiar statement, one I had seen often on buttons, T-shirts and other bumpers before. As a matter of fact, Joan Ullyot has such a bumper sticker. When I once asked her why a woman would display that particular statement, she replied, "It depends on what you mean by *it?*"

But the bumper sticker did identify the owner of that Porsche as a runner. I asked David if he knew the person. "Let's find out," said David, and he pulled his Toyota up even with the Porsche.

The driver of the other car looked unfamiliar to either of us. He seemed middle-aged; he wore a beard. Sitting in the seat beside him was another gentleman, an Oriental. We looked at each other briefly, and for want of anything better to say, I began, "Do you really keep it up longer?"

The driver seemed startled. He did not recognize us either, and I can understand his apparent discomfort. For all he knew, David Pain and I might have been malcontent rednecks who would set upon him with chains for his bumper display. To quickly reassure him, I introduced myself and David. He looked relieved, and recognized our names.

The driver of the Porsche turned out to be Morton H. Pastor, M.D., an anesthesiologist from Coronado. While traffic droned around us, we double-parked and talked. It seems Dr. Pastor had been among 2000 competitors in the Mission Bay Marathon two weeks earlier and, like an angler bragging about a big fish, he talked about finishing the race. It took him four hours and 36 minutes. To put his performance in context, had he been running a course with two laps of 13 miles, Frank Shorter would have lapped him. On my best day, *I* nearly would have lapped him. Yet he was proud of his achievement, and we were proud of him.

"I finished first in my class," announced Dr. Pastor.

"What was that?" David asked.

"First anesthesiologist over 40 who has seven daughters."

As cars behind us honked, and as a traffic policeman stalked suspiciously past, we continued to talk. Dr. Pastor said he began running out of concern for his health. His father died of a heart attack at age 47, and now he had finished his first marathon at the same age, "so maybe I have a better chance." (Indeed, if we believe Dr. Tom Bassler, Dr. Pastor has been granted immunity from a myocardial infarction—as long as he keeps it up!)

He mentioned his mother who nearly three years ago, at age 72, was bedridden, suffering from arthritis and osteoperitis. He put her on a low-salt diet and, after determining there was no underlying serious injury, got her out of bed. She began to hobble around on crutches, painfully at first, then shifted to a cane. Eventually, she threw the cane away and began walking. By the end of a year and a half, she was walking 4-5 miles a day.

He then started her jogging: 30 seconds of jogging followed by a long period of walking, then 30 more seconds of jogging. After one week at that level, she jogged for a minute. This was followed by 10 minutes of walking in between.

"She learned to tolerate this," explained Dr. Pastor, "so we gradually increased the amount of times she would jog and decreased the amount of time walking. Now she jogs 15 minutes four times and walks two minutes in between."

Before beginning on this rehabilitation program, the list of medication being taken by Dr. Pastor's mother included: digitalis, diuretics for congestive heart failure, potassium (to replace that lost with the diuretics), a coronary vasodilator and salt substitutes for her low-salt diet. Bit by bit, he eliminated the medication until the only thing remaining, besides vitamins, was the digitalis. Dr. Pastor said the internist in charge of her case was considering soon eliminating that. During this period of exercise, Dr. Pastor's mother's weight dropped from 155 to 122 pounds. (She is 5'5" tall.)

"Were there any problems?" I asked.

Dr. Pastor thought before he answered. "Yes," he finally replied. "I've had to dye her hair brown. She's going out with younger fellows now."

If there is a lesson to learn from Dr. Pastor, it is this: *When starting a training program, proceed as though it were your aged mother, not yourself, starting to train.* In other words, proceed gradually, one step at a time.

Coincidentally, several weeks later I spoke with another proud son, who taught *his* mother, at age 59, to play tennis. Chuck Sheftel, the teaching professional at the Mid-Town Court House in Chicago, taught tennis for a dozen years before getting involved with the sport of racquetball. He said that three years after his father died, his mother remarried, started a new life and wanted to get active again.

"She played tennis a long time before," explained Chuck, "but once you stop you're in trouble."

He began slowly with her, playing 20 minutes at a time. If he noticed her looking tired, he stopped early. "If you're not used to the game, even holding the racket in your hand for 20 minutes can get tiring," he said.

For the first several weeks, he avoided making her run. Then, gradually, he began hitting the ball to where she would have to take one or two steps to return it. Soon he began hitting the ball two steps to her backhand. At first, his mother admitted a fear of running. Actually, it was a fear of falling. Too many years of inactivity caused her to lose mobility. But soon she actively was playing tennis again.

She continued in that sport, then went through a period when she failed to play for three months. She found herself afraid to start again, the same fear of falling. Chuck resumed the retraining process, but to avoid seeing her lose mobility once more after any more periods of inactivity, he bought her an exercise cycle so she could stay in condition even when not able to get to the tennis courts.

"She bicycles a couple of miles a day now," he said.

Chuck also told the story of having once taught a 75-year-old woman to play tennis, using the same graduated approach. This was in Palm Springs, Calif., and she would arrive at the tennis court in the middle of the day—in fact, in the *heat* of the day—after having played 18 holes of golf with her husband. She told Chuck she was mad at her husband for not playing tennis with her.

"He's just not very athletic," complained the woman.

"How old is your husband?" asked Chuck.

"Eighty-five," she replied.

In summary, both Dr. Pastor's system of teaching his mother jogging and Chuck Sheftel's system of teaching his mother tennis stem from the same philosophy: *You begin very gradually and you always try to achieve less than your potential.*

One of the best progressive forms of achieving fitness was developed by Ransom J. Arthur, M.D. Although designed for swimmers, its pattern easily could be adapted to other similar sports such as running or cycling. Dr. Arthur councils what he calls the "principle of slow induction." By this, he means looking on the program as a long-term commitment. He warns against doing too much exercise too soon.

"This could be dangerous," he advised in an article on Masters swimming. "It should be a matter of months, not days before you swim the full distance you will do in time."

He continued, "More specifically, the first week you might only swim a total of 100 yards each day, broken up into four 25-yard swims, or even less of you have a physical disability. (Many people feel this is too little, but I always counsel patience.) Then, as the weeks pass, gradually increase the amount swum per session. In anywhere from 3-6 months, you'll probably find yourself in pretty good condition and able to swim a minimum of a half-mile at each session (most people can do one mile). People in their 60s and 70s, if fit, are easily able to swim this far. Even a half-mile swim three or four times a week is beneficial."

If you're between 35 and 45, in good health and want to embark on a regular swimming program. Ransom Arthur's is one to follow. Remember that you should embark on this kind of training only *after* your doctor gives you a thorough physical exam *and* his explicit approval to undertake such a program:

First two weeks: swim 100 yards each day in four 25-yard swims.

Next six weeks: swim 200 yards each day in two swims of 100 yards each.

Six weeks to 16 weeks: swim 400 yards each day in three swims of 100 yards each.

Sixteen weeks to 24 weeks: swim 600 yards each day in three swims of 200 yards each.

Twenty-four weeks to 32 weeks: 800 yards each day in either four swims of 200 yards each or two swims of 400 yards each.

At 32 weeks: a minimum of 800 yards a day, either as eight 100 yards, four 200 yards, two 400 yards or one straight 800-yard swim.

Thereafter, you may swim as much more than 800 yards as you wish, but not more than 1 1/2 miles at most. On this program, you should be able to keep your heart, lungs and muscles in excellent condition to the degree that exercise can help.

One important suggestion that Dr. Arthur makes for swimmers is to take a long, hot shower before entering the pool to get their muscles warm and filled with blood. He then advises slow swimming in the early part of the workout before trying any strong swimming. He suggests avoiding all-out sprints. After the workout, he recommends another prolonged shower or sauna bath, followed by a thorough towel-drying to avoid chills.

A period of warmup is advisable for almost all sports, not just swimming. It is particularly necessary if the sport you are about to perform involves sudden movements, yet I rarely see tennis players do what I consider a good warmup before taking racket in hand. If they are wise, they start slowly, hitting the ball back and forth easily, but some do not do that. Chuck Sheftel, in teaching me racquetball, advised a warmup period of about five minutes or so where each player hits the ball easily off the front wall, trying gradually some of the moves he will be required to make later.

"If you are going to have to stretch overhead for a shot during the match," he recommended, "you should make that stretch in your warmups to prepare your muscles."

Of course, with court time costing $9-12 an hour players may be tempted to squeeze as much play as possible out of their hour. If so, they should do their stretching in the hall outside the court before their hour begins.

I have acted in the summer theater and often I would warmup before taking center stage by doing the same exercises I used prepatory to running a track race. Some of the other actors looked at me strangely, but if nothing else the exercises helped relax me so I would not forget my lines. In musicals, our vocal coach always recommended we warm up our voices before trying to hit any high notes.

A good period of stretching is also a good insurance policy against injuries. I once heard a story about a track coach on the

East Coast whose team constantly seemed plagued by injuries. He learned of a doctor with a good reputation for treating athletic injuries and brought one of his team members in for a visit. The doctor recommended stretching exercises for the runner. The coach thanked him, left, and because several years passed without any more contact between the two, the doctor assumed the track coach disliked his advice and went to another doctor. Then one day he met the coach on the street and asked him about the matter.

The coach explained, "I started everybody on the team doing the stretching exercises you suggested. We just don't have many more injuries."

Stretching exercises have become very much the vogue among world-class athletes. Rich Wohlhuter, 800-meter bronze medalist in the Olympics at Montreal, constantly was bothered by achilles tendon injuries while in college at Notre Dame. This severely restricted his ability to compete. In his last few years of college, however, working with his coach, Alex Wilson, he developed a series of stretching exercises, the simplest one being to lean forehead against the wall with his feet several feet away from the wall and his heels flat on the floor. By use of this simple stretching exercise, Rick almost completely eliminated his previous tendon troubles and soon set world records for 880 yards and 1000 meters.

Flexibility is extremely important if you want to both avoid injuries and run fast. (Fast for a jogger might mean eight-minute mile pace; everything is relative to both your ability and point of view.) As a result, many runners I know are into yoga. At Runner's Mecca, one of the most pleasant parts of each day was the yoga class taught each morning by Bruce Gove, a coach from Upland, Calif. For someone who wants to learn yoga at home, the book *Light On Yoga* has an excellent set of exercises.

I never will have the flexibility of either my wife and daughter, who can sit on the floor and almost press their foreheads to the ground. I am content merely to be able to touch my toes, something I had lost the ability to do until convinced by Roy Benson, distance coach at the University of Florida and director of the Florida Distance Camp, that stretching could improve my ability to run faster. (Long-distance runners have a tendency to lose flexibility by running distances at slow paces on hard ground.)

There is a secret to touching your toes, as Roy Benson convinced me. Bouncing up and down in a calisthenic-like toe-touching exercise sometimes tightens the muscles more than it loosens them. Roy preached the "Hang 10," where you simply lean forward and let your 10 fingers dangle toward your toes. If you do not rush things, you should sooner or later be able to touch them. It took me about six months (not continuous activity, of course!).

I find I can get still lower if I stretch up before I reach down. I stand feet together and reach with my arms over my head, trying to stretch as far as I can, not only in my shoulders but through my stomach muscles. Then I gently tip forward and reach for the floor. Remember: don't bounce.

Several yoga exercises can be performed while standing up. Bruce particularly stressed these in his classes, because it is easier for runners to start a long workout on the roads, then pause at about one mile for several minutes of stretching before continuing down the road. I am convinced that any distance runner or jogger who does this will not only improve his flexibility but will limit his injuries as well.

I also am convinced that the same would be true for individuals in other sports—for example, tennis. A good rule for tennis players would be to jog several times around the courts before they play, then do some stretching. They would find themselves better warmed up, but they probably would improve their cardiovascular fitness as well. A few more laps around the court after each match probably would lessen the impact of stiff muscles, particularly for weekend athletes.

One of my sons, David, is in a "junior excellence" program at the Northwest Racquet Club, an indoor tennis facility near our home. He goes twice a week for practice sessions and also competes for the club team. On several occasions I have driven him to workouts and stayed long enough to notice that the coach puts team members through running drills. If running is good for actively competitive players, it should be equally good for social players. In fact, social players may benefit more from it.

The danger of injury increases in almost any fitness sport when an individual becomes very competitive about that sport, especially if that person is middle-aged or older.

"My training has always been interrupted by injury," David

Pain admitted to me. "And many Master athletes have that same problem. That causes dropouts, because guys who are potentially fine athletes just plain give up. They start training, get in shape and injure themselves before a key meet. Finally, they say, 'The hell with it!' and go back either to doing nothing or get involved in some other sport."

If the latter is the case, then they probably lose little, because men and women past 40 do not need to engage in competitive programs to keep physically fit. They merely need to remain active. What is the minimum amount of exercise an individual needs in order to maintain fitness?

Chuck Sheftel offers some common-sense words of advice: "Once a week is not enough," he advises. "You have to break a sweat at least three days a week for 20 minutes each time. That's when you're in shape."

Bill Bowerman, former track coach from the University of Oregon, utilized a pattern that always appealed to me in my training. Bowerman would alternate his charges in hard days and easy days. They would run extremely hard on one day, take a relatively easy workout the next, then be rested enough so they could go hard again on the third. Of course, the amount of effort that went into one of Bowerman's "easy" days would put the average weekend warrior in bed until the next weekend, but the pattern of hard/easy/hard/easy remains the most sensible approach to training I know. I use this pattern, so do most of the better distance runners I know, and it is eminently adaptable to other sports such as swimming, cycling or tennis.

Considering the schedule limitations of most people with business careers, I would modify it slightly to accommodate those weekend warriors who wage athletic battles on weekends simply because that is the only time that they have sufficient time for much athletic activity. Maybe it is too much to expect everyone to get out for an hour of physical activity every day of the week, but it should be possible to get out on alternating days. This suggests a four-days-to-fitness schedule something like this:

Saturday: three sets of aggressive tennis.
Sunday: two hours of cycling in the park.

Monday: total rest to recuperate from weekend excesses.
Tuesday: a half-hour swim at the YMCA.
Wednesday: more rest.
Thursday: 2-3 miles of easy jogging.
Friday: rest to store up energy for the weekend athletic wars.

The individual who follows a schedule like that might never become world champion or even club champion, but he would remain physically fit. Depending on how much effort went into each of those days, I suspect he would come close to scoring the 30 Aerobics points that Dr. Kenneth Cooper identifies as the threshold of fitness.

Some of us are fortunate enough to be adept at a sport, such as running, that seems to offer optimum physical benefits while satisfying our craving for both competition and sociability. But it is possible to live a Marathon Life Style without being a marathon runner. Marathon Life Style relates as much to diet, sleep and enthusiasm for life as to any particular athletic discipline. Many tennis or handball players who never run more than three successive steps may have Marathon Life Styles without realizing it.

For those who seek fitness and do not have one sport, I suggest you not worry about it. Instead, do as I described in Chapter 13 and become Renaissance Sportsmen; seek many athletic disciplines. When the snow falls, ski. When the snow melts, jog. When the melted snow warms, swim. When the lake cools, cycle. When it finally freezes, ice skate. Enjoy life. Enjoy living.

Despite what you may have heard from others, there is no easy route to total fitness. You cannot get in shape on five minutes a day. You will not become physically fit by exercising a half-hour a week. You may achieve a better level of fitness than the person who does nothing, but that is a small accomplishment.

Even if we accept Dr. Tom Bassler's assertion that finishing a marathon provides immunity from heart attack, that person is not granted immunity for life. Dr. Bassler concedes that the immunity fades once a person discontinues his Marathon Life Style. This is true regardless of your sport. Gains are temporary.

The secret, then, if you want to maintain good health for the rest of your life, is: *keep it up.*

Epilogue:
How to Live to Be 99

The question of how long a person will live resists easy answer. Whether or not you will be alive next year depends, first, on whether you are here this year. Life may be blotted out at any moment, for almost any reason. Many fetuses never see the light of day, victims of abortion. Other babies die during the struggle of birth. The leading cause of death among young people is accidents, mostly in automobiles. People die of drug overdoses.

If we fail to die of such unnatural causes, various natural causes will kill us: heart disease, cancer and what some people refer to as simply old age. There is no precise way of predicting when you will go. The ground may open beneath your feet any minute—particularly if you live along the San Andreas Fault. Of course, you could always move to another area of the country—and be swept up in a tornado or drowned in a flood. Life is precious to each of us, but with four billion people on this planet (give or take a few million) and many thousands of them dying every day, it is statistically unprecious.

However, it is also statistically predictable. By examining life insurance actuarial tables and considering some of the risk factors of life as determined by researchers such as Dr. Herman K. Hellerstein, it is possible to project the possibilities of longevity.

For example, census figures in the United States indicate that a white male that reaches the age of 45 will live to the age of 72-plus years. Life expectancy for most women is higher, with a white female of the above age projected to live six years longer. If you are black, however, your life expectancy is significantly lower. The life expectancy for most non-whites at birth averages six years less than whites, although by age 65 the differences almost even out.

Ignoring, for the time being, both sexual and racial differences, the following chart (utilizing both census data and Metropolitan Life Insurance Company statistics) offers a beginning to predicting whether you will live to be 99 or longer. If you have reached the number of years indicated in the first column (age), you should live to be as old as the number in the second column (expectancy).

Age	Expectancy	Age	Expectancy	Age	Expectancy
30	74	44	75	57	78
31	74	45	76	58	78
32	74	46	76	59	78
33	74	47	76	60	78
34	74	48	76	61	79
35	74	49	76	62	79
36	74	50	76	63	79
37	75	51	77	64	79
38	75	52	77	65	80
39	75	53	77	66	80
40	75	54	77	67	80
41	75	55	77	68	81
42	75	56	77	69	81
43	75			70	82

But the above life expectancy chart only *suggests*, unprecisely, how much longer the *average* person will live having reached a certain age. Anyone reading a copy of this book presumably is *above average*, because of your obvious interest in health and fitness. If you also are above average in your habits and heredity, you will live still longer. Those below average die sooner.

Various methods can be used to project, with some reliability, a particular individual's longevity. Several years ago, author Judith Bentley devised a test entitled "Will You Live to Be 100?" which appeared in the January 1975 issue of *Family Health*. It later was adapted by Dr. Diana S. Woodruff of Temple University into a test entitled "How to Pass the Test of Time," which appeared (among other places) in the *Chicago Tribune* of Jan. 23, 1977.

This was gamesmanship at its best. I could prove how fit I was and be the first person in my block to know my date of death. Taking the Woodruff test, I projected my life expectancy at 88 years. Some time later, I uncovered and took the Bentley test and learned I would reach 91. (Bentley determined her own life expectancy at 79; Woodruff did not announce hers.)

The existence of such tests opened interesting possibilities. If I only could continue to find newer and better life expectancy tests, I might continue to increase the possibilities of my living a fuller and better life. So rather than leave that to chance, and the whims of magazine and newspaper editors, I decided to devise a longevity test of my own, utilizing some of the ideas of Woodruff and Bentley, while applying the knowledge gleaned while writing this book. The resulting Higdon Test follows. Perhaps you would like to take it along with me to see who will outlast the other.

1. Expectancy. Consult the chart at left. We are going to figure in points rather than years, so depending on your present age you will score the number of points equal to the number in the expectancy column opposite your age.

I am 45, so I earn 76 points for having survived this long.

My score   76   *Your score* _____

2. Heredity/parents. Did your mother and father live past age 70? If so, chances are you will, too. Add one point for every five-year period per individual. But this is a double-edged sword: If your parents died younger than that age, and it was not an accident-related death (such as an automobile crash), subtract one point per five-year period.

My father died of a heart attack at age 69. My mother remains alive at age 80. I receive two points, but the scorebook on this section, for me, remains open.

My score   78   *Your score* _____

3. Heredity/grandparents. If your grandparents lived past 80, add one point for every five-year period per individual; younger than 60, subtract one point per 10-year period..

My grandfathers died relatively young, and for reasons of which I am not certain. However, my grandmothers exhibited remarkable longevity. One lived to age 86, the other to 94. I earn three points for them, but lose an equal number because of my grandfathers dying in their 40s and 50s.

My score   78   *Your score* _____

3. Heredity/medical. If any of your parents, grandparents, brothers or sisters died of a heart attack or stroke before the age of 60, subtract two points. Subtract two more points if before the age of 50, and continue to penalize yourself for each 10-year increment. If any of those relatives have, or had, diabetes, thyroid disorder, cancer, asthma, emphysema or chronic bursitis, penalize yourself three points for each incident.

As far as I know, none of the above relate to me, but I do have hay fever (inherited from my mother), so I'm accepting one penalty point.

My score   77   *Your score* _____

4. Sex. If you are female, score three points. If you are a male, subtract three points. Women live longer than men. A 30-year old male has a life expectancy of 70.9 years compared to 77.3 years for his female counterpart. Even at age 70, the male-female expectancy ratios are 80.4 and 83.6 years, respectively.

However, if you are a liberated female occupying a job, forget it. You blew your advantage, baby. Subtract one point. If that job is one previously held almost exclusively by males, subtract two points. If you carry a membership card in the National Organization of Women, or have lobbied for equal rights, subtract three points. Did you think freedom comes without a price?

As a liberated male, I lose three points along with my sisters.

My score   74   *Your score* _____

5. *Race.* If you are black, you will live a shorter life than most whites, as mentioned earlier. Although the life expectancy difference between black and white children at birth is six years, much of this is because of factors covered elsewhere in this test, such as heredity, diet and social status. Subtract two points if you are black and under 35; one point, if black and under 60.

Being white, I stay even.

My score   74   *Your score*_____

6. *Diet.* If you weigh too much, subtract one point for every 10 pounds of excess fat. Too much blubber puts an unnecessary strain on your heart and limits your mobility, which is also a factor in mortality. Pay no attention to what the medical height-weight charts say, since they offer only vague guidelines and can vary by 30-40 pounds depending on so-called frame-type. But *you* know what would be an ideal weight for you if you avoided those cookies in the pantry. Don't cheat.

I stand 5'10" tall and now weigh 145 pounds, somewhat heavy for optimum efficiency as a competitive long-distance runner but not too far above the 142 pounds which I consider best for myself as a human being. I earn no penalty.

My score   74   *Your score*_____

7. *Alcohol.* If you normally consume two drinks or more a day (whether cocktail, beer or wine), subtract one point for every drink-per-day you sink toward alcoholism. If you are a moderate drinker (1-2 a day), no penalty; if an occasional drinker (1-2 a week), accept one point.

Woodruff and Bentley penalized teetotalers one point on the theory that non-drinkers have rigid value systems and may undergo stress in maintaining them. I disagree, but even if true, penalties for that personality trait would appear elsewhere in this test. If you never, and I mean *never*, touch a drink I'll give you two points on merit. (There is a history of alcoholism in one branch of my family, so perhaps I am oversensitive as to the dangers of excessive drinking.)

As a now-and-then drinker, who has an occasional beer (with popcorn) while watching TV movies and who shares a half-liter of wine with my wife when we eat dinner out, I'll modestly accept one point.

My score   75   Your score_____

8. Sleep. If you stay in bed nine hours daily, subtract three points. If more than 10 hours, penalize yourself six. The theory here is that individuals who sleep that much spend too many hours involved in non-physical activity, either because of weakness or as an escape. If you sleep *less* than six hours a day, take two points off for each hour less. You probably work too hard and get insufficient rest.

I fall in that happy middle area. Usually during the week, I go to bed around 11 or 11:30 p.m. and rise by 6 or 6:30 a.m. But there is a positive factor in my favor coming up.

My score   75   Your score_____

9. Naps. Both Woodruff and Bentley overlooked this category. If you supplement your night's sleep with a short nap of at least 4-5 days weekly, add one point for each day. Remember, I said *short* nap. If you stay on the couch longer than an hour, or if your nap pushes your sleep total past nine hours, you receive no credit. Napping is an efficient way of regaining energy, particularly right after a meal. Many parents, who insist their young children take naps, probably should accept their own advice.

I am a nap-taker. Give me four points. Because I work at home, I have the freedom to nap any time of the day, so usually I rest for a half-hour immediately after lunch, then return to the typewriter refreshed. One good friend of mine, travel writer Dick Dunlop, says if he feels tired he stops to nap any time of the day, and several times a day. But when 5 p.m. comes, he quits work—whether or not he has had enough sleep.

My score   79   Your score_____

10. Physical examination. Women older than 30 who give themselves monthly breast examinations add one point, provided you also have an annual physical examination with a Pap smear. Men older than 40 who have an annual physical that includes a proctoscopic examination (to detect cancer of the bowels), add one. If the physical examinations include a stress test at least every other year, add one more point.

I have not had a proctoscopic examination, perhaps because of being lulled into security by the treadmill tests that I undergo frequently at various physiological labs. But I am claiming one point for regular stress tests.

My score   80   *Your score*_____

11. Cigarettes. Prepare yourself for a lecture. If you smoke up to 10 cigarettes a day, subtract two points. If you smoke one pack a day, subtract two more points. If you smoke more than one pack, subtract two additional points per pack. (It is not merely the threat of lung cancer, it is coronary artery disease, emphysema, lack of mobility and more.)

And this may surprise you: If you work in an area where your fellow workers smoke around you, or if your wife or husband smokes, subtract two points. Don't protest to me; protest to them. It isn't enough merely not to smoke; you also have to avoid nicotine addicts, since you will find yourself breathing their exhaled air. Blood tests have shown that a person who works in an office with heavy smokers also absorbs nicotine into his system. That person may inhale the equivalent of 4-8 cigarettes a day without realizing it. If this makes you mad at smokers, it should.

If your parents smoked while you were a child, what I am about to say may also turn you against them. If your father, or particularly your mother, smoked indoors near you during your first six months of life, this probably stigmatized you for life and limited your potential as an athlete in endurance events.

The lungs of newborn children are particularly pliable during this six-month period and will rapidly absorb nicotine from the air. If you happened to be born during the winter, you probably suffered more damage to your pulmonary system because of being forced to remain in the house more. Summer-born children suffer fewer dibilitating effects to their maximum oxygen potential, according to Dr. Tom Bassler. He suggests that a future long-distance runner with smoking parents loses six minutes from his potential marathon time for each month (of his first six months of life) spent mostly indoors.

Therefore, if you are a non-smoker who neither lives nor works with smokers, add two points. If you ever have asked an individual not to smoke in your presence, add two more points. (You may lose those points later for having a Type A personality, but we'll get to that.)

I am a militant non-smoker, becoming more militant every day. While waiting to appear on a television talk show to promote a race in Gainesville, Fla., I noticed a symphony musician also scheduled for the show pull a pack of cigarettes from his pocket. Without saying why, I stood and left the room, to be followed at five-second intervals by Dr. Joan Ullyot and race director (and runner) Nick West. They knew my reason for leaving. Later, when I mentioned that incident during a lecture that night, the audience broke out in applause.

Many non-smokers, like I, have learned the dangers of indirect inhalation, and we accept our four points with malice and fists raised in the air.

My score   84   *Your score* _____

12. Exercise. If you exercise three or four times a week, score two points. If the amount of exercise you get is sufficient to score 30-35 points on Dr. Kenneth Cooper's Aerobics charts, add two more points. If you exercise *only* on weekends, subtract two points. You may be doing yourself more harm than good by subjecting your heart to sudden stress without proper preparation.

I earn four points, the maximum, but get no extra bonus because of the excessive exercise I get as a competitive runner.

My score   88   *Your score* _____

13. Marathon. Dr. Tom Bassler suggests immunity from heart attack to those adopting the "Marathon Life Style" and finishing a 26-mile, 385-yard marathon. If this is you, accept three more points, provided you trained a minimum of one year to run your first race longer than 10 miles and started that race with no interest in the time you finished. If you ever participated in a long bicycle touring trip (minimum: 75 miles) or have participated (rather than competed) in any similar endurance activity, with gradual preparation similar to that undertaken by back-of-the-pack marathoners, you also may claim three points.

My first attempt at the marathon was at Boston, and I ran with the leaders until they left me, then dropped out soon after. I was more interested in winning than finishing. It took me four attempts before I finally got to the finish line in a marathon. I eventually placed fifth at Boston, running 2:21:55 in 1964, but while I have a magnificent trophy in my bookcase, it will not help me live longer. No more points.

My score 88 *Your score* _____

14. Marital status. If you are married, add three points, since married people live longer. If single, through choice or divorce, subtract one point for every year of age past 30. If you are living with a member of the opposite sex and are unmarried, subtract two points. At least, that's what Ann Landers told me to tell you.

As a husband and father of three, I score three points, one per child, although that is coincidental. Mothers with more than that number should probably begin subtracting points.

My score 91 *Your score* _____

15. Type A. If you bound out of bed early every morning, get upset when your spouse is late and like to dominate conversations, you have what Dr. Meyer Friedman described in his book as a Type A personality. Most successful competitive athletes probably have Type A traits, confidence and desire being major factors in athletic success.

If you must be dynamited out of bed by a jarring alarm clock each morning, are the spouse who is always late and enjoy sitting back at large gatherings so you can observe others, you fit the Type B mold. Most joggers, who care not how fast they run but only that they run, could be considered Type B. Rate yourself on a scale of 1-5 as either A or B. If you are the former, subtract that number of points. If the latter, add the appropriate amount.

As a runner, I can be extremely competitive at times. I do bound out of bed every morning and often am sitting in the car drumming my fingers on the steering wheel waiting for my wife to come downstairs. But at other times, I enjoy the luxury of going for a long run at no particular speed for the pure enjoyment of it. Like many runners, I suspect I fluctuate between Type A and

Type B traits, depending on my mood. But score two negative points for the former.

My score   89   *Your score*_____

16. Safety. If you refuse to put your car in gear without fastening your seat belt, add one point. If you also busy yourself digging the belts out from under the cushions while a passenger in someone else's car, add two. If you buckle up only occasionally, subtract one. If you think safety belts such a nuisance you never use them, subtract two.

The death toll from traffic accidents each year in the United States is 50,000. Having written enough articles on traffic safety to know the odds, I am fanatic about using safety belts. I snap them on even to drive two blocks at 20 m.p.h., and snap at my family if they fail to wear them. I gain back those two points I lost for having a Type A personality.

My score   91   *Your score*_____

17. Education. If you graduated from high school, add one point. If you graduated from college, add one more. If you attended graduate school, add still another. The better educated you are, the more likely are you to understand the importance of health care in prolonging life. You also probably earn more money and have access to better health care.

Bentley and Woodruff suggested that anyone making over $40,000 probably suffers more stress and consumes richer food, but Dr. Hellerstein indicates that the opposite is true. Lower-income people suffer more stress and compensate by eating more food, and the wrong kind of food. If you fit this last pattern—less than 10 years of education, low income—subtract three.

Having attended graduate school, I'm claiming two points.

My score   93   *Your score* _____

18. Social status. Dr. Hellerstein also determined that parents, regardless of background, who earned good salaries and attained relatively high status, raised their children to have better health habits than themselves. If your parents were members of the upper middle class, score one point. If not, subtract one point.

My father never graduated from grade school, but he pulled

himself up by his bootstraps in order to give me a better life before he died of a heart attack. I accept one point in his memory.

My score   94   *Your score*_____

19. Happiness. Rate the level of your happiness on a scale of 1-5. Give yourself the appropriate number of points.

I love my wife. I love my three children. I love my job. I love to run. Give me one point for each of the above. If I could think of something else, I would really be happy.

My score   98   *Your score*_____

20. Attitude toward fitness. If you cared enough about your own health to purchase a copy of this book, score two points. If you borrowed it from a friend or the library, you score only one point. If you are the author of the book, that is worth one point.

Some might consider this cheating, but I take points where I can get them. I claim my final score.

My score   99   *Your score*_____

Each point you score is worth one year of longevity. If my calculations prove correct, and if the above system is valid, I shall live to be 99 years old. When I took the test prepared by Woodward and Bentley, I scored 91 and 88 points respectively, proving there may be no value in any of our tests. If you failed to score as many points as I did, keep watching the obituary columns for my name. You still may have the last laugh.

Acknowledgements

Fitness After Forty is my 17th book in a writing career that began in 1959 when I left my job as assistant editor on *The Kiwanis Magazine* to see if I could make a living as a free lance writer. When I originally supplied dust jacket copy for this volume, I said 15 previous books, but recounted and found one more. They have varied in subject matter from history to business to crime to sports.

In most of these books, I have eschewed the ordinary author's acknowlegements. My theory was that acknowlegements mostly are a form of padding, written to salve the author's ego and as a means of offering thanks to people who should have been thanked personally. I always disliked reading laundry lists of source people, so assumed others (except for those who made the list) disliked reading them, too.

Nevertheless, for *Fitness After Forty* I have received more than the usual support and feel obligated to offer public thanks. I still do not want to offer the usual laundry list of source people, since their names are scattered throughout the book. It does not take much imagination to discover that people such as Dave Costill, Marc Sorenson and Ken Cooper (to name only a few) provided me with assistance and information. Often, when I found myself stymied for some particular piece of information, I picked up the telephone and obtained an authoritative answer almost instantly, from them or from others.

But there are others whose assistance may not be quite so apparent. For example, Hortense Leon of Chicago, served as a researcher for *Fitness After Forty* and provided the basic information that resulted in the first chapter about how the human body deteriorates. And Ken Young of the National Running Data Center (although previously credited) designed the many statistical charts dealing with that same subject at my request. Ivan Fuldauer, a public relations gentleman from Chicago, otherwise invisible, assisted me in gathering data related to racquetball and related sports. Joseph Breu on the news staff of the American Medical Association aided my interviews.

Katie Foehl, news bureau manager for Presbyterian-St. Luke's Hospital, helped make arrangements connected with the coronary bypass chapter, then suffered with me when the physicians involved insisted they wanted no publicity because they feared censure from their medical colleagues for "advertising" (thus the one pseudonymous physician in that chapter). Theodore Berland, a fellow member of the American Society of Journalists and Authors and writer of a regular diet column in the *Chicago Daily News*, served as a consultant on the section of the book dealing with diet.

Valerie Brady transcribed the many tape-recorded interviews I did with the source people in this book and assisted with typing, along with Rosanne Campagna and Maryann McKenna.

And although they provided no direct input for *Fitness After Forty*, I also should mention my wife Rose and my three children Kevin, David, and Laura. They put up with me amidst trying times, particularly during the last six weeks of writing when I was working 12-14 hours daily trying to meet a tight deadline. (I use my wife as a consultant on most of my writing, asking her to read early drafts to see if they are any good, then getting mad at her when she says they are not.)

My running during this trying pre-publication period deteriorated to two miles daily and I suffered withdrawal symptoms. I slept fitfully, feeling pains in my chest and arm which I felt certain were symptoms of an impending heart attack. I overate. My weight soared to 145, 10 pounds over my racing best. It occurred to me during this frantic period that I might write a book on fitness which would extend the lives of thousands of Americans, while shortening my own. I knew any royalties earned would soon by squandered to pay for a coronary bypass operation.

Joe Henderson, editor of *Runner's World*, also served as editor of this book and helped make sense out of it. He is author of an impressive five-foot shelf of books on running that any serious runner has read, or *should* read, and I felt honored to have him. Joe and I first met soon after I got out of the Army and was running for the University of Chicago Track Club. It was 1959. He was a bright and eager high school kid from Iowa who traveled all the way into Chicago for our summer all-comer meets. Joe claims he ran in a 3000-meter steeplechase against myself and Mike Manley (then also in high school, later an Olympian). He claims I won. I hate to think of defeating people. I would much rather remember the Petaluma Marathon several years ago where Joe and I crossed the finish line in a tie. Our friendship continues.

But possibly the one individual who has had the greatest impact on this book, who will share in any success it attains, is Bob Anderson, founder of *Runner's World* and director of World Publications. I wrote an article for one of the first issues of the then-called *Distance Running News*, back when Bob was an eager high school kid from Kansas.

The effect Bob has had on *Fitness After Forty* can best be explained by mentioning that when I originally proposed the book to him, the title was *Fitness Man Meets the Aerobic Monster, or How to Run the 100-Yard Dash at Age 98*. I'm serious. I was thinking of a book on Masters running that would mainly be humorous, in the tradition of my previous *On the Run from Dogs and People*. That book, for all its celebrity among long-distance runners, sold only 3000 copies. Nobody owns a copy of that book. Anyone who ever read it either borrowed it from a friend or took it out of their local library.

Bob felt that our new book should be instructive and include all fitness activities for older people, not just running. That he was right is evident from the first printing order of 25,000 copies for this book, necessitated by advance orders.

Let me say a word before closing about John Blackburn, M.D., father of Jack Blackburn, whom I ran against in the 10,000 meters at the 1956 Olympic Trials. Jack later switched to race walking and several years later I helped officiate a National AAU 20 or 25 kilometer walk in which he, as well as his father, participated. I was then in my 20s, and after the race I looked at Dr. Blackburn, a man in is 40s, shirtless because of the heat, trim, lean, youthful, vigorous. I thought, "When I'm his age I want to look like that."

I think I succeeded, and if everyone who picks up a copy of *Fitness After Forty* (whether from a friend or a library) heeds its message, they can, too.

—Hal Higdon